54693A

3600

9988

THE TEAM APPROACH
TO HEMIPLEGIA

THE TEAM APPROACH
TO HEMIPLEGIA

Edited by

CHARLES D. BONNER, M.D., D.Sc. (Hon.), F.A.C.P.

Director, Cardinal Cushing Rehabilitation Center
Holy Ghost Hospital
Cambridge, Massachusetts
Assistant Clinical Professor of Medicine
Boston University School of Medicine
Boston, Massachusetts
Lecturer in Physical Medicine and Rehabilitation
Tufts University Medical School
Boston, Massachusetts

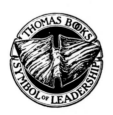

CHARLES C THOMAS • **PUBLISHER**
Springfield • Illinois • U.S.A.

Published and Distributed Throughout the World by
CHARLES C THOMAS • PUBLISHER
Bannerstone House
301-327 East Lawrence Avenue, Springfield, Illinois, U.S.A.
Natchez Plantation House
735 North Atlantic Boulevard, Fort Lauderdale, Florida, U.S.A.

With THOMAS BOOKS *careful attention is given to all details of
manufacturing and design. It is the Publisher's desire to present books
that are satisfactory as to their physical qualities and artistic possibilities
and appropriate for their particular use.* THOMAS BOOKS *will be true
to those laws of quality that assure a good name and good will.*

Printed in the United States of America
W-2

CONTRIBUTORS

STAFF

Joanne C. MacDonald, M.A., O.T.R.
Former Supervisor, Occupational Therapy
Cardinal Cushing Rehabilitation Center
Assistant Professor, Occupational Therapy
Boston University

Elizabeth F. Morris, M.S.W.
Director of Social Service
Cardinal Cushing Rehabilitation Center

Adrienne H. Nelson, B.S., R.P.T.
Former Staff Physical Therapist
Cardinal Cushing Rehabilitation Center

Barbara Z. O'Neill, M.Ed.
Speech Therapist
Cardinal Cushing Rehabilitation Center

Meribah E. Stanton, B.S., R.N.
Former Rehabilitation Nurse Supervisor
Cardinal Cushing Rehabilitation Center
Instructor of Nursing
Quinsigamond Community College

GUEST

Norman R. Bernstein, M.D.
Assistant Director, Child Psychiatry
Massachusetts General Hospital
Boston, Massachusetts
Director, Psychiatric Training Program
Walter E. Fernald School
Waltham, Massachusetts

Theresa DePippo, M.P.H.
Public Health Nutrition Supervisor
Division of Adult Health
Massachusetts Department of Public Health

Harold Goodglass, Ph.D.
Chief, Clinical Psychology Section
Veterans Administration Hospital
Boston, Massachusetts

Francis A. Harding
Former Commissioner
Massachusetts Rehabilitation Commission

This book is dedicated to my mother and all other stroke patients who were stricken and disabled and who died without the benefit of dynamic physical restoration. Their collective misfortune inspired my intense concern and a personal commitment to provide an adequate treatment program for as many stroke patients as my human capabilities would permit.

PREFACE

 $\mathbf{F}$ OR MANY YEARS people who suffered cerebral vascular accidents were relegated to a life of inactivity and neglect. These patients were routinely treated by bed rest, general nursing and custodial care. They were frequently considered as unexciting and unnecessary admissions to general hospitals and were rapidly referred for transfer to nursing homes, to chronic hospitals or to the community. Mortality and morbidity were high.

Since World War II the field of physical medicine and rehabilitation has enjoyed a renaissance. A new dynamic approach making possible the restoration of the cerebral vascular accident patient to his maximum level of potential independence in all spheres has been developed. Now some of these individuals are receiving the type of active management comparable to that which is provided in other areas of modern medicine. However, in spite of the advent of this "third phase of medicine" and the establishment of many rehabilitation centers throughout the country, the vast majority of these patients still do not receive adequate care and/or comprehensive management.

For the stroke patient who has a spontaneous recovery or for the stroke patient who expires at the time of the accident, this poses no problem. For the hundreds of thousands of other stroke patients who are left with varying degrees of physical disability, their whole future is at stake. It is unfortunate that the apathy shown toward stroke patients by most of those responsible for their care continued to be of such magnitude that a President's Commission was established and the ground work for federal involvement to assure more adequate care for the cerebral vascular accident patient became necessary.

It is encouraging that many groups today, especially the paramedical groups, are taking an intense interest in caring for the stroke patient, and are looking to physicians for leadership. It is hoped that the physician in turn will become more enthusiastic about this problem and accept his role of leadership unflinchingly and with more aggressiveness.

Eighty per cent of all disabled cerebral vascular accident patients can become independently ambulatory and/or independent in activities of daily living. Fifteen to 20 per cent can return to productivity in the work field. All can enjoy better health through better care. It is therefore hoped that this book will offer specific and general guidance to those who desire to provide more adequate management for their stroke patients.

CHARLES D. BONNER

ACKNOWLEDGMENTS

THE AUTHOR WISHES to express his sincere appreciation to Miss Mary Jane Arrigo for typing this manuscript in its multiple phases. The extra hours invested, numerous revisions made and tired fingers endured displayed a dedication beyond the call of duty.

Thanks are also extended to James F. Townsend, P.S.A., and his wife Kathleen, a member of our physical therapy staff, for the excellent photographs included in the book.

Additional thanks must be given to Miss Bernice Lyford, R.P.T., Miss Charlene Pehoski, O.T.R., Miss Barbara Gannon, R.N., and Mrs. Frances Physic, R.N., for their helpful suggestions and criticisms.

The cooperation of the patients and staff members who allowed themselves to be photographed is also deeply appreciated.

The services of Mrs. Susie Jones in reviewing the galley proofs were of great value.

The moral support offered and patience demonstrated by wife, Frances, and daughters, Carol and Dale, during the preparation of this manuscript is acknowledged with the deepest gratitude.

C. D. B.

CONTENTS

THE TEAM APPROACH
TO HEMIPLEGIA

Chapter I

PHILOSOPHICAL APPROACH TO THE CARE OF THE STROKE PATIENT

TWENTY YEARS AGO

NOTHING DISTURBED THE elderly man, sleeping so peacefully in his bed at three o'clock one morning, nothing alerted him to the fact that only a few feet away, C. B., his 64-year-old wife, lay helpless on the floor, unable to move her right arm and leg, her power of speech completely gone.

A few minutes earlier, C. B., who never before had experienced any difficulty in getting out of bed, awakened for one of her several nightly trips to the bathroom. This time, however, something was wrong! With great difficulty she moved to the side of the bed and laboriously pulled herself to a sitting position. It was when she attempted to stand that she fell to the floor where for seemingly endless hours she lay in the dark, frightened and alone in the stark realization of her plight. When her husband finally awoke, missed her in bed, and found her paralyzed and speechless, he somehow managed to get her back into bed. Then another disturbing discovery was made—she could not control her bladder and she wet herself.

When the family physician examined C. B., about seven o'clock that morning he stated categorically that the patient had suffered a cerebral hemorrhage; nothing could be done for her, and she must stay in bed. As the physician prepared to leave, C. B. felt the need to urinate and not wanting to wet herself again, tried to get up. The physician immediately pushed her back, told her not to get out of bed under any circumstances, and instructed the family to restrain her if necessary. A neurologist from a medical school faculty, called in for further consultation, concurred with the family physician and dogmatically

3

stated that nothing could be done for this patient other than to give her the routine nursing care that any family could offer.

TEN YEARS AGO

When 70-year-old J. C. suffered a cerebral hemorrhage which paralyzed her left side, she was admitted as a bed patient to a general hospital. Here, despite the fact that she had three special nurses around the clock, she was placed on catheter drainage. After six weeks she was transferred to a chronic disease hospital for rehabilitation where the concept of self-care at its lowest level, that of feeding herself, was introduced. Although J. C. had no coordination difficulty in her unaffected arm, she had become so accustomed to being fed by the nurses that she refused to cooperate. Her family, at first strenuously opposed to her being asked to feed herself, was amazed when it was pointed out that since the patient had one good arm there was no valid reason why she shouldn't use it to help herself. However, J. C., caught in her own motivationless web, pressured the family so heavily that against their better judgment they took her home. There she was again put to bed and made a permanent, chronic invalid, destined for an earlier death than might otherwise have been expected.

SIX YEARS AGO

In a paper entitled "Prognostic Evaluation for Rehabilitation of Patients with Strokes," one of us (Dr. Charles D. Bonner) wrote as follows:

> Current experience with restorative treatment of hemiplegic patients indicates that, despite the growing acceptance of rehabilitation concepts and the establishment of rehabilitation centers throughout the country, physicians still need practical information on the prognostic evaluation of stroke patients with varied degrees of physical and mental incapacity. This need for information is documented by the following incidents.
>
> Firstly, personal discussions with medical students during the course of medical teaching revealed that the majority have had no contact with a rehabilitation unit and actually have no idea of the high degree of independence which a stroke victim can attain.
>
> Second, during a recent visit in a medical ward of a large

teaching hospital, six patients who had experienced cerebral thromboses with hemiparesis within the preceding six weeks were awaiting
disposition to nursing homes without receiving or being considered
for rehabilitation therapy. The house staff had assumed that nothing
could be done for them.

Third, a senior medical resident, when instructed to refer a
hemiplegic patient for rehabilitation, stated that in all of his medical
training he had never been taught anything about the rehabilitation
of such patients and he did not realize their potential for physical
independence. Further a chief resident of a neurologic service, when
called in consultation to see a patient with interesting neurologic
findings resulting from a cerebral thrombosis, stated that the opportune time to begin mobilizing the patient would be three to four
weeks after the inception of his stroke. The patient, even at the
time of consultation, was showing return of function in the affected
extremities and had initiated a request to be permitted out of bed.

Fourth, many questions asked and statements made by lay
people with hemiplegic relatives revealed that most of them had
been told by their family physicians that nothing could be done for
this type of patient and that they should either plan to care for the
patient at home or arrange for his transfer to a nursing home. This
unenlightened attitude has been confirmed by personal discussions
with practicing physicians and is further attested to by the fact that
the Holy Ghost Hospital, Rehabilitation Center, which is the only
facility of its kind in a community of 100,000 population, received
only six applications for the treatment of stroke patients from the
doctors and hospitals of the community during the past five years—
this in spite of 200 stroke patient admissions per year to the local
general hospitals.

Despite the encouraging trend toward more widespread
acceptance and application of rehabilitation techniques, the
above cases and situations unfortunately, but accurately, reflect
the attitudes of many individuals who become involved in the
care of aged, chronically ill patients. Pessimism, misunderstand-
ing, conservatism, skepticism, and lack of knowledge are the rule.
And standing in the shadow of these misapprehensions is the
stroke patient—helpless, desperate, needing skilled assistance
more than ever before in his life.

It is a sad commentary that such conditions exist in what is
presumably one of the most enlightened periods of American
history, especially in view of a constantly rising life expectancy.
During the past century enormous strides have been made in

finding the cause, control, or cure of many of the medical problems which contributed to the high death rate of times past. Two thousand years ago the lifespan of the average human was 25 years. At the turn of our century this had increased to 49 years, and today life expectancy is between 71 and 74 years of age in countries where modern methods of medical practice are applied. It is somewhat difficult for some of us to realize that there are still areas of the world where modern medications are not available, hunger is rampant, and the life expectancy is still only approximately 45 years.

In 1900, older people made up 4 per cent of the population, whereas today almost 9 per cent fall into this category. Furthermore, among the aged, the proportion at the extreme ages is also rising. In 1940, 30 per cent of the United States population 65 years of age and over, were at least 75 years old; today, more than 35 per cent of these senior citizens are in this group. More than 10,000 Americans are 100 years of age or older. This represents a fivefold increase in the older population during the twentieth century, an increase brought about by such discoveries as insulin, which controls diabetes; penicillin and broad-spectrum antibiotics, which cure many formerly critical bacterial infections; antituberculosis drugs, which are stamping out this scourge; various hormones, which are controlling endocrinological problems, as well as preventing debility; and new and advanced methods of surgery, among which reconstructive and cardiac repair are the most spectacular. The Salk polio vaccine has proved itself 90 per cent effective in preventing paralytic forms of this disease, and many other vaccines prevent diseases which were highly fatal in years gone by.

While these statistics are encouraging, they also indicate that the constantly increasing medical problems which we face in this expanding population of the aged are those caused by severe crippling trauma, neurological conditions, and degenerative disease. In 1957, the United States National Health Survey reported that approximately 38 per cent of our population under age 65 suffered from some form of chronic ailment, while in the group which included persons age 65 and older, 83 per cent (more than twice the number of the younger group) reported at least some chronic condition. To add to the seriousness of the problem of chronic illness in our aged population, the number of chronic conditions per aged patient is also more than double that of the younger patient.

In the forefront of this aging population with many chronic problems stand the stroke patients, two million strong, hoping for a better chance.

Therefore, one may legitimately ask, "Why should such waste be permitted? Why do we fail to utilize to the fullest extent the excellent medical care and facilities which exist and which *are* available for the dynamic care of the stroke patient?" Without the benefit of these advantages, these ailing, incapacitated old-sters may look forward only to enforced inactivity, decreased job opportunities, reduced income, lower standards of living, and ultimate rejection by society. There should, can, and *must* be a brighter outlook for these countless unfortunates.

Happily, concrete means for achieving this goal are within the reach of medical and paramedical personnel alike, and these will be discussed in detail in the following chapters. However, there are less apparent but equally important attributes involved in the care of chronically ill persons and the following five suggestions are presented as a means for providing a more knowledgeable approach to intelligent care:

1. Awareness of the patient's mental and physical capa-bilities is vital. For instance, one should know that most stroke patients who are able to understand simple directions can be retrained to dress, feed, and bathe themselves, tend to their own toilet needs, and to walk. Further, one must be aware of the preventive techniques designed to avert secondary complica-tions and of the availability of the services provided by medical and paramedical personnel, therapists, and agencies created to give financial aid.

2. Knowledge of where and how to locate these services is a must. It should be emphasized that passive acceptance of nursing care alone is not enough; rather, the person entrusted with the patient's care must be constantly alert to the possibility of the patient's actual potential and make a concentrated effort to foster this potential by rapid and proper referral.

3. A bit of daring should be injected into a proposed therapeutic program since generally accepted, conservative methods of management often fail to provide the patient with the necessary tools for maximum recovery. There should be no hesitation in trying new approaches, new mechanisms of action, modern equipment, and improved therapies. One need only remind himself that failure to make a bold approach may spell the difference between the patient's recovery and shattered hopes.

4. Faith, which sometimes accomplishes the seemingly impossible, is another essential factor in caring for these patients and it must be twofold. The person involved in patient care must have faith in both himself and in his patient. Confidence in one's knowledge, skill, tolerance, and tenacity of purpose will be communicated to the patient who in turn will develop motivation, will put forth the effort to improve, and eventually will achieve his goal. Thus, faith which nurtures *hope* becomes a precious commodity in the life of the invalid and must be made an integral part of the program.

5. Above all, the capacity to love, and the ability to express this love, are requisites to providing total care of the highest order. The patient who suddenly comes face to face with himself in this new role of the helpless invalid suffers severe emotional shock. Now weak, seemingly alone, and above all, frightened, he must reconstruct his relationship to family, friends and society. He is at the lowest ebb in his life and his behavioral pattern is often at its worst. He needs love and understanding desperately, and those striving to work successfully with him must offer not only all the technical skill at their command, but also more affection and understanding than they believed they possessed. They must project a shining goal, never accepting defeat in its pursuit, and by so doing, love in the strictest sense of the word will be expressed.

FOUR MONTHS AGO

Four days after P. G., a 61-year-old man, suffered a coronary occlusion, he developed paralysis of the right arm and leg and loss of speech. After one month as a bed patient in a university teaching hospital where he was given anticoagulants and supportive therapy, the patient was transferred to a hospital for chronic diseases with the prognosis that he would never walk again. In accordance with the teaching hospital's recommendation, P. G. was admitted to the custodial section of the chronic disease hospital for terminal care. However, after his history had been recorded and a physical examination made, he was referred to the rehabilitation division for evaluation. This revealed dense paralysis of the right arm and leg and the inability to speak. However, a redeeming factor was P. G.'s ability to follow simple directions, and he was accepted into the rehabilitation program. Despite the fact that the patient had a half-inch separation of his right shoulder which limited shoulder motion and caused considerable pain, a four-point program was set up for him: (1) to mobilize the affected shoulder; (2) to maintain the full range of motion in the paralyzed arm and leg; (3) to reorient him to an upright position, and (4) to make him ambulatory. Also planned were occupational and speech therapy, the former to complement his work in physical therapy and to retrain him for activities of daily living; the latter to improve his ability to communicate, if possible. P. G. made fairly rapid physical progress. He soon became accustomed to the upright position and advanced to the parallel bars for gait training. (It must be noted that all this was accomplished without the return of function to his right arm.) He was fitted with a short-leg brace and, over a period of a month and a half, learned to walk with a cane; he also learned to dress himself. P. G. was discharged from the hospital, going home to a newly acquired first-floor apartment from which he continued his speech therapy on an outpatient basis at the rehabilitation center. Today he is completely independent in all daily living activities.

The above story relates the happy conclusion to a situation which had a sad but usual beginning. We must all pressure for active stroke care programs throughout the nation so that each afflicted individual will have an equal opportunity to write his own success story with as happy, or even happier an ending than that of P. G.

The care of cerebral vascular accident patients can be one of life's most satisfying endeavors, provided a dynamic, searching approach is made by those entrusted with this care. It is at this crossroad that the individuals destined for oblivion, the difficult cases, the so-called crocks, etc., can through adequate management follow the proper pathway back to society as independent participants once again.

REFERENCES

BONNER, C. D.: Prognostic evaluation for rehabilitation of patients with strokes. *Geriatrics, 14*:424, 1959.

Facts on Major Killing and Crippling Diseases in the United States Today. The National Health Education Committee, Inc., 1961.

HOMBURGER, F., AND BONNER, C. D.: *The Medical Care and Rehabilitation of the Aged and Chronically Ill.* Boston, Little, 1965.

Chapter II

THE CHARACTERISTICS OF STROKE PATIENTS AND THE IMAGE THEY CREATE

Old Lady And The Rubber Ball*

She looked down at her hand. There was a rubber ball in it. Somebody said softly: "Squeeze it." She tried. Her dark brown eyes watched gravely as the fingertips fluttered. The Old Lady could not squeeze. The hand was palm-up on her thigh. The ball looked like a red eye in a wrinkled socket. She was dreaming.

Not dreaming. She could smell the antisepsis in the room, and the Old Lady had never smelled anything in a dream. It was real. She was sick. The mass of tangled black and white hair lifted up, and the brown eyes looked around the room slowly, slowly. Beds. Many beds.

The Old Lady understood. But how did she get here? What happened? She tried to reconstruct. Thoughts tumbled down the rapids of her mind, but they were too fast. Someone said softly: "Squeeze it" and she looked down again and willed the fingers to close over the ball. They declined the order.

She felt no pain. Nor fear. Confusion, yes. For the first time, the Old Lady noticed that she was in a wheelchair. She looked at her knees, and saw that she was wearing a gray bathrobe. She was in some institution. A ward. She had had an accident. Or a heart attack. Or a stroke. Yes, a stroke. That was it.

The grave eyes turned on the doctor crouched before her. "Docker," her mouth said, "plee temmee . . . ." She heard the croaking voice. Fear squeezed the heart. She could not speak properly. Could . . . not . . . speak. She wanted to say: "Doctor, please tell me . . ." but the words fell from the sagging mouth awkwardly.

The Old Lady began to weep. There was no sound. The blinking brown eyes squeezed the tears off. The young doctor stood. "She

------

* Reproduced with the permission of Jim Bishop, Reporter, from the Saturday, April 10, 1965 issue of the *San Francisco Examiner*.

11

knows," he said to himself. "For the first time, she knows." He patted the lifeless hand, and left. He had other work.

The Old Lady was there a long time. She and the rubber ball became inseparable. Her speech improved, but the fingers remained divorced. She was a charity case, but this did not hurt. She felt that she had always been a charity case.

One day her nephew stopped in. He was young and dark and wholesome to study. He told her how great she looked, and not to worry, she would be out of here in no time. The crooked mouth smiled.

After fifteen minutes, he began to study his watch. He frowned. She understood. She looked at the tall lean figure, and tried to commit it to memory. He was such a good boy. Always thoughtful.

She watched him reach into his pocket and saw the ten-dollar bill. He grinned. "I'll leave it in your night table," he said. "It's for tips." She shook her head no. "Come on," he said. "For bobby pins. A smidge of lipstick." No, she said. No.

The Old Lady formed the words slowly, "If . . you . . want . . to . . leave . . the . . money," the brown eyes swung across the room, "leave . . it . . with . . that . . old . . woman . . who . . has . . the . . bedclothes . . over . . her . . head." The nephew looked. "She . . has . . asked . . to . . go . . home. They had . . to . . tell . . her. She . . has . . a . . married . . daughter, and . . they . . don't . . want . . her . . back."

"Poor . . thing. She . . cries . . all . . the . . time." The nephew shrugged. "Who is your friend?" he said. The brown eyes looked down at a hand. The Old Lady had the rubber ball. . . .

The major reason the stroke patient is treated with such indifference by the medical fraternity is the negative image which has been perpetuated throughout the years. The stroke patient has always been reluctantly admitted to most hospitals and often even before adequate investigation has been completed, active referral has been made for rapid disposition. The above article typically represents the image many people have of this type of patient. The afflicted Old Lady with a mass of unkempt tangled black and white hair sat in the wheelchair by herself with a typical institutional type grey bathrobe in a room of many beds. The doctor came, uselessly because he knew (mistakenly) that nothing could be done, patted her lifeless hand and left because he had other work to do. By this action he also successfully conveyed to the patient that her condition was hopeless. Words fell from her sagging mouth awarkedly and without intent; she began to weep. The blinking brown eyes squeezed the tears off. Her nephew visited, and in fifteen minutes he was ready to go. His guilt was assuaged by depositing a ten-dollar bill on the bedside table for incidentals. And through it all the old lady had, the rubber ball, a symbol to many people of therapy for a weakened hand which in reality creates more in the way of complications than benefits.

These patients are usually found in bed. They are usually poorly groomed with hair uncombed, faces unshaven, dentures in a jar on the table rather than in the mouth, thus sagging cheeks and dressed in depersonalized hospital johnnies which permit little privacy should the patients be out of bed. If the affected side has a significant degree of remaining paralysis, the arm is usually drawn up into a flexion pattern which may be accentuated by spasticity. The lower extremity may also be contracted. In many instances this type of patient receives inadequate amounts of fluid resulting in a bone-dry tongue, a fetid odor to the breath because of poor oral hygiene, and mental confusion. There is usually the inevitable, unnecessary urethral catheter hanging over the side of the bed into the open drainage bottle. Unfortunately, the patient is frequently left waiting in bed for that day in the future (which may never come) when by some miracle he will arise and walk without anyone's assistance.

It is therefore time to exchange this routine unattractive image for a true image of hope. With the incorporation of many old, but sound methods of physical restoration, plus the addition of many newer modern dynamic techniques, and with the availability of many rehabilitation centers, physical therapy departments in acute hospitals, and home programs, the stroke patient can be brought back to a useful life.

It must be realized that all stroke patients are not old. Many individuals in the younger age group suffer strokes because of ruptured aneurysms with extension of subarachnoid bleeding into the brain substance. Other younger people with rheumatic heart disease and auricular fibrillation may have embolic phenomena to the cerebral vessels. Not uncommonly, individuals in their forties are seen who have actual thromboses. These may be in the form of plaques in the carotid system, but pathological sections of brains have been viewed of people in their forties where the cerebral vessels were as arteriosclerotic as those of a 70-year old. Many of these patients are young mothers and fathers with family responsibilities. Therefore the vision of the stroke patient as always being an oldster is not accurate, and many of these younger individuals and certainly many older ones as well have a great deal of potential, not only for life, but for return to the labor and professional market.

The results of only basic grooming can be amazing. Patients have been seen in general hospitals in consultation who at first glance fitted the description of the old image above. Following acceptance to our rehabilitation center and the admission to our rehabilitation ward, these patients become completely different individuals within twenty-four hours, and often unrecognizable as the same people. This positive transformation was brought about simply by having their hair neatly combed or styled; perhaps a colorful ribbon was placed in the hair of a woman; the patients' dentures were in their mouths and a tub bath had been given. Further, the patients were wearing their own clothing, including colorful blouses, shirts, slacks, socks and shoes; the catheters had been removed and they were sitting up in a wheelchair as part of a living group. No therapy at this point had been instituted, but human dignity had been restored and created a new spark of life in eager eyes. Immediately they were allowed to do the things for themselves which they could, and often for the first time they were brushing their own teeth, washing their own faces and upper torsos, and they were taken to the bathroom where they had privacy, rather than the bedpan. They were only assisted in and out of bed, but did most of it themselves, and for the first time they had hope and felt suddenly like human beings again rather than hopeless victims destined to a living death.

There are no rubber balls in these hands to assist in making flexion contractures. These patients are involved in a dynamic program of increasing muscle strength, learning to stand and transfer, improving balance, becoming proficient in activities of daily living, and eventually walking. They can feel the strength of many potentialities surge back into their very beings. And after experiencing such a comprehensive program for a varied length of time, these patients are ready for discharge back into the community, not only as part of a family group, but as contributing members of this group and at times even as wage earners again.

This is the type of image we must create for the stroke patient. This degree of independence in walking, in activities of daily living, and in working can be achieved for most of them if they are given the opportunity. If we routinely saw this image in our mind's eye rather than the old lady with the rubber ball, more stroke patients would be rescued from the pangs of depression and loneliness which have been their lot in the past.

Chapter III

ETIOLOGY

T HE MATERIAL TO be presented in this chapter is not meant to be a detailed discussion of subject matter which is more elaborately described in other textbooks. However, it will serve to orient the beginner and it may serve to correct some misconceptions which seem to be present in the minds of some physicians.

The term *cerebrovascular* includes all diseases in which one or more blood vessels of the brain are primarily involved in a pathological process. An abnormality of the vascular wall, occlusion by thrombus or embollus, change in the caliber of lumen, and altered permeability to plasma and blood cells would all be grouped under this term.

The outline below is a classification of cerebrovascular disease reported by an *ad hoc* committee of the Advisory Council for the National Institute of Neurological Diseases and Blindness of the Public Health Service. The main basis of the classification is pathology except in those disease categories where only clinical features are known.

    1. Cerebral infarction (pale, red hemorrhagic and mixed types)
      A. Thrombosis with atherosclerosis
      B. Cerebral embolism
        1. Of cardiac origin
          a. Atrial fibrillation and other arrhythmias (with rheumatic, arterosclerotic, hypertensive, congenital heart disease)
          b. Myocardial infarction with mural thrombus
          c. Acute and subacute bacterial endocarditis
          d. Heart disease without arrhythmia or mural thrombus
          e. Complications of cardiac surgery
          f. Nonbacterial thrombotic ("marantic") endocardial vegetations
          g. Paradoxical embolism with congenital heart disease

    2. Of noncardiac origin
       a. Atherosclerosis of aorta and carotid arteries (mural thrombus, atheromatous material)
       b. From sites of cerebral artery thrombosis
       c. Thrombus in pulmonary veins
       d. Fat
       e. Tumor
       f. Air
       g. Complications of neck and thoracic surgery
       h. Miscellaneous: rare types
       i. Of undetermined origin
  C. Other conditions causing cerebral infarction
    1. Cerebral venous thrombosis
    2. Systemic hypotension
    3. Complications of arteriography
    4. Arteritis (see VI)
    5. Hematologic disorders (polycythemia, sickle-cell disease, thrombotic thrombopenia, etc.)
    6. Dissecting aortic aneurysm
    7. Trauma to carotid
    8. Anoxia
    9. Radioactive or x-ray radiation
   10. With tentorial, foramen magnum, and subfalcial herniations
   11. Miscellaneous: rare types
  D. Cerebral infarctions of undetermined cause
II. Transient cerebral ischemia without infarction
  A. Recurrent focal cerebral ischemic attacks (Previously called vasospasm, usually associated with thrombosis and atherosclerosis)
  B. Systemic hypotension ("simple faint," acute blood loss, myocardial infarction, Stokes-Adams syndrome, traumatic and surgical shock, sensitive carotid sinus, severe postural hypotension)
    1. With Focal Neurological deficit
    2. With syncope
  C. Migraine
III. Intracranial hemorrhage (Including intracerebral, subarachnoid, ventricular, rarely, subdural)
  A. Hypertensive intracerebral hemorrhage
  B. Ruptured saccular aneurysm (If unruptured See IV A)
  C. Angioma (If unruptured See IV B)
  D. Trauma
  E. Hemorrhagic disorders (leukemia, aplastic anemia, thrombopenic purpura, liver disease, complication of anticoagulant therapy, etc.)
  F. Of undetermined cause (normal blood pressure and no angioma)

G. Hemorrhage into primary and secondary brain tumors

H. Septic embolism, mycotic aneurysm

I. With hemorrhagic infarction, arterial or venous (see under I and VII)

J. Secondary brainstem hemorrhage (temporal lobe herniation)

K. Hypertensive encephalopathy

L. Idiopathic brain purpura

M. With inflammatory disease of arteries and veins (see under VI, VII)

N. Miscellaneous: rare types

IV. Vascular malformations and developmental abnormalities

A. Aneurysm—saccular, fusiform, globular, diffuse (if ruptured see III B)

B. Angioma (including familial telangiectasis, trigeminal encephalo-angiomatosis [Struge-Weber-Dimitri], retinal-pontine hemangiomas) (if ruptured see III C)

C. Absence, hypoplasia, or other abnormality of vessels (including variations in pattern of circle of Willis)

V. Inflammatory diseases of arteries

A. Infections and infestations

1. Meningovascular syphilis

2. Septic embolism

3. Arteritis secondary to pyogenic and tuberculous meningitis

4. Rare types (typhus, schistosomiasis mansoni, malaria, trichinosis, etc.)

B. Diseases of undetermined origin

1. Lupus erythematosus

2. Rheumatic arteritis

3. Polyarteritis nodosa (necrotizing and granulomatous forms)

4. Cranial arteritis (temporal)

5. Idiopathic granulomatous arteritis of aorta and its major branches

VI. Vascular diseases without changes in the brain

A. Atherosclerosis

B. Hypertension arterio- and arteriolosclerosis

C. Hyaline arterio- and arteriolosclerosis

D. Calcification and ferruginization of vessels

E. Capillary sclerosis, etc.

VII. Hypertensive encephalopathy

A. Malignant hypertension (essential, chronic renal disease, pheochromocytoma, etc.)

B. Acute glomerulonephritis

C. Eclampsia

VIII. Dural sinus and cerebral venous thrombosis

A. Secondary to infection of ear, paranasal sinus, face, or other

       cranial structures
- B.   With meningitis and subdural empyema
- C.   Debilitating states (marantic)
- D.   Postpartum
- E.   Postoperative
- F.   Hematologic disease (polycythemia, sickle-cell disease)
- G.   Cardiac failure and congestive heart disease
- H.   Miscellaneous: rare types
- I.   Of undetermined cause
- IX. Strokes of undetermined origin

Of the nine groupings above, the first three include the types of strokes seen most frequently. Focal arterial disease of the brain can also be classified into three stages by the clinical status of the patient.

These three stages are defined as impending or incipient stroke, progressing stroke, and completed stroke. In the first stage, brief, transient episodes of neurological dysfunction take place, but the status of the patient returns to normality in between. During the second stage, the neurologic deficit continues to progress or gets worse while still in the early phase of symptomatology. The completed stroke has reached its maximum neurological deficit, has been stable for hours or days, and then may begin to show improvement.

The most common type of cerebral vascular accident is caused by a thrombosis of one of the arterial systems involved in supplying blood to the cerebral hemispheres. At one time such strokes were thought to only occur in the cerebral arteries themselves. With modern techniques, however, it has been possible to demonstrate that thromboses take place not only in these arteries but also in the basilar-vertebral arterial system, the circle of Willis, within the carotid artery near its bifurcation and in its immediate branches. The thrombotic phenomenon may be represented by extensive arterial involvement whereby long segments of arteries are occluded with calcific and fatty deposits or by one plaque strategically placed at a narrow point of passage.

Disease of the cerebral vessels themselves is usually heralded by a singular episode which may be slow in onset. The patient may be left with complete or partial paralysis or may recover.

Disease in the basilar-vertebral system or carotid tree however may create symptoms at first which are transient and minor. These should serve as a warning of more serious problems to come and stimulate investigation of the cause.

It is not enough to make the diagnosis of thrombosis. The specific site should be determined if possible because some lesions lend themselves to surgical removal or bypass grafts while others may be alleviated by anticoagulant therapy. The arrival at a correct diagnosis and the institution of appropriate active treatment may prevent major neurological residual.

Obstruction in the carotid arteries is heralded by a bruit, grade 1-4, which can be heard by stethoscope when placed over the artery. This diagnostic procedure has not received sufficient recognition within the medical profession and should be incorporated into the regular routine of all physical examinations. The presence of a bruit plus transient symptoms should stimulate immediate investigation and definitive treatment.

Patients who suffer from strokes caused by cerebral emboli usually fall into the younger age group. This disease is primarily secondary to heart disease with atrial fibrillation but can also be caused by other cardiac disorders such as bacterial endocarditis, mural thrombus following myocardial infarction, cardiac surgery or by fat, tumors, and air. With modern methods of arrhythmia control and anticoagulation, the incidence of this type of accident is diminishing. However, frequently the anticoagulation procedure or the attempt at rhythm conversion takes place after the embolus has occurred and initial damage has been done.

Subarachnoid hemorrhages are also a cause for strokes in a certain percentage of patients so afflicted. The severity of this condition can vary from the patient who ruptures an aneurysm and develops no neurological deficit to the patient who dies. In between is the patient whose aneurysm ruptures out of the subarachnoid space and into brain substance. Correct location of the aneurysm is vital as it may be possible to obliterate it surgically and prevent further bleeding episodes. Many are located in the circle of Willis but other arteries are also commonly involved. Some patients can have more than one aneurysm present, all or any combination of which can rupture. Not all locations lend themselves to surgical intervention.

The frank intracerebral hemorrhage is usually caused by a significant elevation of blood pressure and in the majority of cases results in death. Of those who survive many have experienced such massive cerebral damage that they are unable to cooperate in any rehabilitation process. However, a small percentage of this group will still have significant potential for rehabilitation and this potential should be utilized.

The above four entities include the most frequent causes of cerebral vascular accidents. There are other processes which can damage the same areas of the brain and result in similar strokelike syndromes. Included among these is trauma such as caused by automobile accidents, falls from heights, blows from blunt objects, etc.; expanding lesions, both benign and malignant; vascular inflammatory diseases and hematological disorders. Intracerebral hematomas are also found in younger people, secondary to bleeding of undetermined etiology.

Although the etiology of the cerebral vascular accident can be quite varied and require a different type of preventive measure for each, the residual physical disability is similar and the team approach to the rehabilitation of the individual applies.

REFERENCES

A classification and outline of cerebrovascular diseases. A report by an *ad hoc* committee established by the Advisory Council for the National Institute of Neurological Diseases and Blindness, Public Health Service. *Neurology,* 8:5, 1958.

MILLIKAN, C. H.; SIEKERT, R. G., AND WHISNANT, J. P.: *Cerebral Vascular Diseases* (Third Conference). New York, Grune, 1961.

Chapter IV

NOMENCLATURE

One of the weakest links between referring physician and rehabilitation center is the characteristic use by the former of nonspecific terms as they relate to the stroke patient. Ninety per cent of the referral blanks have such nondescript diagnoses as "CVA," "left hemiplegia," "cerebral hemorrhage," "stroke," etc. In most instances very little additional descriptive information is furnished. The reviewing physician frequently has to reject the application or send for additional information before he feels secure in accepting the patient into the hospital. Otherwise a physician evaluation in the referring hospital is necessary or the patient must be brought to the rehabilitation center for evaluation and then sent back to the referring hospital if rejected or to await a bed.

The outline below is suggested to encourage the use of more specific terms by physicians. It will accomplish several useful purposes if used as a guide. For instance, primarily and foremost it will dispel the idea that all stroke patients are the same. If one takes the time to fill out a referral form by this outline and subsequently compares a number of them, he will see that most stroke patients are quite different. They may present a similar overall problem, but each also presents specific individual problems. This outline will therefore give the physician a much clearer idea of the diversity of problems of his own patients. Second, it will give the reviewing authority in the rehabilitation center concrete data to study which will help in making the decision concerning admission to the center or rejection.

A. *Etiology*

This item is self-explanatory and has been covered in Chapter

22

III. Knowledge of the precise etiology of the stroke is helpful not only in the prevention of further disease, but in establishing possible prognosis. One should state whether it has been caused by a thrombosis, embollus, hemorrhage, subarachnoid hemorrhage or other cause (see Table I).

B. Arterial System Involved

With the advent of surgical techniques which can alleviate certain specific lesions and the use of anticoagulants which may prevent further clot formation it becomes necessary if possible to pinpoint the actual arterial system which is involved. In this way strokes cease being just ordinary strokes and create an investigative challenge. Location of the lesion in the cerebral arteries, in the carotids or in the basilar vertebral system should be made.

C. Mental Status

This is one of the most important items requiring accurate description. The patient must have enough mental alertness and receptive cerebration to understand, to follow simple commands, and to cooperate in a progressive rehabilitation program. Ability to remember instructions from day to day is desirable, but it should be emphasized that many patients who have slight impaired cerebration with mild confusion or memory defect still can meet this minimal requirement and often achieve successful final results. The patient who cannot relate or respond to stimuli of this type and who is unable to cooperate should not be referred for an active program.

D. Side of Peripheral Manifestation

The side or sides involved should be stated. This knowledge also has some prognostic importance, as patients with left-sided involvement often tend to be unaware of their affected side and seem subject to deeper depression. Patients with involvement of their right side more frequently have speech problems, though this is not an absolute finding.

E. Degree of Paralysis

The functional capacity of the involved extremities is often

TABLE I

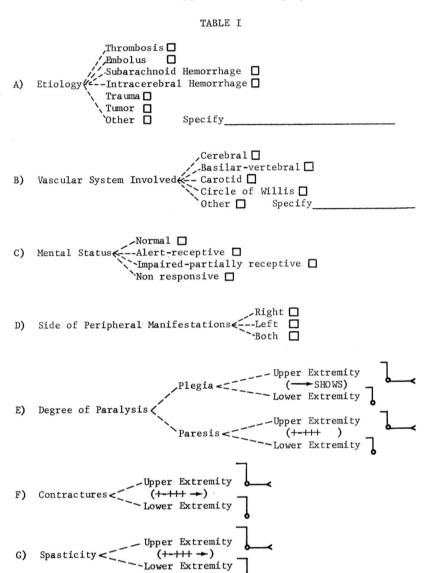

A physician should fill out this outline for each disabled stroke patient. It will provide a factual summary of the problems of each patient which will not only assist the physician in determining prognosis but will also be of inestimable value to other agencies who may later be responsible for the patient's care.

TABLE I (continued)

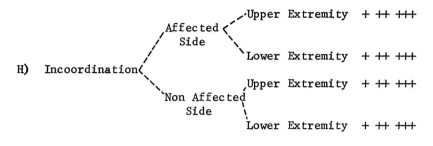

H) Incoordination

Affected Side
- Upper Extremity + ++ +++
- Lower Extremity + ++ +++

Non Affected Side
- Upper Extremity + ++ +++
- Lower Extremity + ++ +++

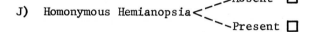

I) Sensory Deficit ⟵ — — Absent ☐
Present ☐
(+-+++ ⟶)

J) Homonymous Hemianopsia
- Absent ☐
- Present ☐

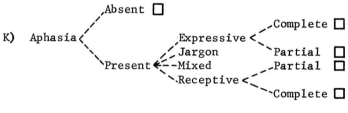

K) Aphasia
- Absent ☐
- Present
  - Expressive
    - Complete ☐
    - Partial ☐
  - Jargon
  - Mixed
  - Receptive
    - Partial ☐
    - Complete ☐

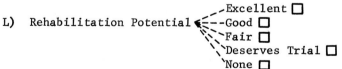

L) Rehabilitation Potential
- Excellent ☐
- Good ☐
- Fair ☐
- Deserves Trial ☐
- None ☐

⟶ Area Involved
+ ++ +++   Slight   Moderate   Severe   Involvement

misstated. In many instances the patient is called "hemiplegic" and this word is used as a blanket term. It frequently includes patients who do have return of active motion in their affected extremities, and it does not depict the patient whose upper extremity may be paralyzed, but whose lower extremity may demonstrate some active return of function. It is therefore suggested that paralyzed upper and lower extremities be designated as plegic and weak ones as paretic. A simple line diagram with small arrows can be used to designate the actual muscle groups which are plegic or paretic as shown in Table I. In a paretic extremity the use of simple line diagrams and arrows with a 1+ to 3+ evaluation can be used to show the actual degree of strength which is present in each described area.

F. Contractures

Unfortunately many patients are still referred to rehabilitation centers without having received preventive measures of treatment. Fifty to 60 per cent of these patients arrive with contractures involving the upper extremity, usually the shoulder, wrist, and fingers; and 25 to 35 per cent show some degree of contracture of the lower extremities, usually the ankle and knee. Since this is a very important factor in the ultimate prognosis, prior knowledge of this information would be most helpful. Again by using simple line diagrams and arrows with 1+ to 3+ designation, the area of the contracture and its degree of severity can be documented.

G. Spasticity

Most patients who suffer a cerebrovascular accident will develop some degree of spasticity in their involved extremities as muscle power returns. This at times relates to the ultimate functional ability the patient may receive. The upper extremity is more severely involved in most instances and frequently it remains a functionless extremity. The lower extremity is involved, but usually to a lesser degree and there have been few instances where spasticity has been the primary factor in the patient not becoming ambulatory. This factor may also be demonstrated by the use of simple line drawings and the use of arrows with 1+ to 3+ designation of the actual muscle groups involved.

H. Incoordination

This is a less common finding, but its presence is important in the overall prognosis. It may not be of great importance in the affected upper extremity which has inadequate hand function, but in the restored hand it interferes with fine dexterity. It is of more significance when it involves the so called non-affected upper extremity because this is often the one which the patient is dependent upon to replace the abilities missing from the affected extremity. Its presence and degree of severity can be denoted by circling the appropriate 1+ to 3+ group on the outline.

I. Sensory Deficit

The presence of a sensory deficit is most important if heat modalities are to be utilized. Also if the patient may be exposed to open radiators, pipes, smoking or matches, etc., it is vital information to have. Its presence may be denoted with a simple line drawing pointing out the area involved and the degree of involvement. This will insure extra caution in the use of hot packs, heat lamps, paraffin dip, etc., by the therapists.

J. Homonymous Hemianopsia

The presence of this deficit has many important implications. It should be considered in the proper placement of a patient in the nursing unit so that his available vision is directed towards the overall center of activity. Bedside table, water pitcher, food tray, etc., should be placed on the side of the patient's active vision. Those who take care of the patient must be aware of the problem and approach the patient from this same direction if they expect the patient to work up to his best potential.

K. Aphasia

For the patient this may be the most frustrating area of his disability. A complete understanding of this deficit must be had by all members of the rehabilitation team. It is therefore important to know whether aphasia is present, whether it is expressive and complete or partial, whether it is jargon type or mixed, or whether there is a complete or partial receptive

characteristic. This again can help determine the patient's
probable potential.

TABLE II

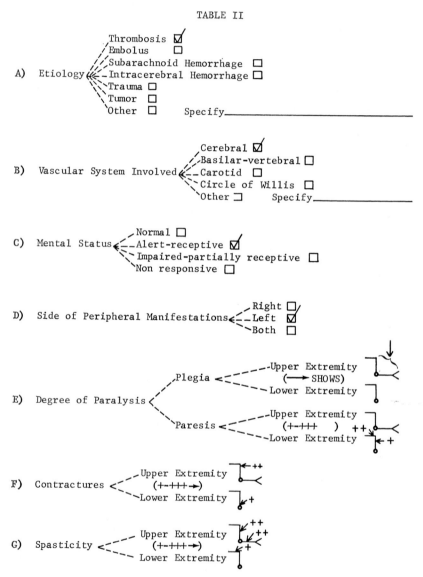

A sample copy of the above suggested outline which has been filled out for
a specific patient (see text).

L. *Rehabilitation Potential*

The referring physician should finally indicate on the outline just what he thinks about the patient's potential. This is another way in which the plight of the stroke patient may be progressively improved. The physician must go through the mental

TABLE II (continued)

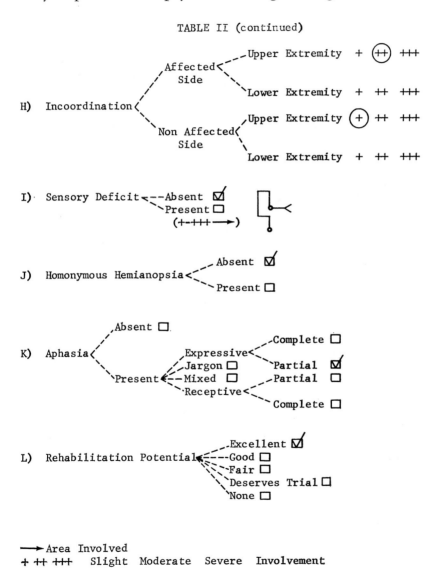

→ Area Involved
+ ++ +++   Slight Moderate Severe Involvement

process of adding up all the positive and negative values demonstrated in the above outline and then make up his own mind whether he thinks the patient will make a good candidate or not. His opinion can later be checked against the actual final result achieved after treatment in the rehabilitation center and a continuous educational process will ensue. Below is an example of how the outline might work in an actual situation (see Table II).

A 62 year-old female is being referred for possible admission to a rehabilitation program. The diagnosis of cerebral thrombosis has been substantiated and located in the right middle cerebral artery. Her mental status is alert, receptive, and cooperative, and the peripheral side involved is the left. There is a complete left upper monoplegia and a left lower monoparesis with no motion in the foot. There is a moderate contracture of the shoulder and a slight contracture of the ankle. There is moderate spasticity in some muscle groups of the upper extremity and slight spasticity in the lower extremity. Moderate incoordination is noted in the upper extremity of the affected side and slight incoordination in the upper extremity of the nonaffected side. There is no sensory deficit present and visual abilities are intact. A partial expressive aphasia is present. In this patient the potential for rehabilitation is considered to be excellent.

The use of this outline should bring the problems of the stroke patient into better focus. It will not only help the referring physician in his assessment of his patient, but the physician in the rehabilitation center who must decide which patients his services will best benefit. However, the people who will benefit most by the mental procedures involved in completing this outline will be the stroke patients themselves who finally will no longer be classified as just hopeless stroke patients, but patients whose individual potentials add up to positive prognostic signposts.

Chapter V

CONFERENCE TECHNIQUE

W HEN A STROKE occurs, the patient usually consults a physician. Although cerebral vascular accidents take place at any time or place and under many possible circumstances, the patient is usually seen by his own physician, by an emergency physician, or taken by ambulance or car to the emergency room of his community hospital.

When it is time for referral to a formal rehabilitation program, the patient requires an assessment of his deficits and potentials. This assessment varies depending upon the staff organization of individual rehabilitation programs. Rehabilitation centers which are affiliated with chronic disease hospitals lend themselves to the use of the conference technique of evaluation. Patients admitted to such centers have been referred from general hospitals or private physicians and have had their medical workups completed. An objective evaluation of liabilities and assets can therefore be performed within a reasonable amount of time.

In the rehabilitation center at the Holy Ghost Hospital a specific time is set aside weekly when all team members sit together in one large conference and see and participate in the evaluation of all new patients who will soon be under their active care. All members of the physical, occupational, and speech therapy departments attend, as well as all social workers, all nurses who may be released from the ward at that time, and all students who are at that moment affiliated with or assigned to any of the above departments.

This technique has stimulated so much interest throughout the community that at almost every session guests from surrounding hospitals or teaching institutions are present who wish to observe the team approach to hemiplegia in action. This conference has also been attended by many individuals from other

31

countries, and the universal feeling expressed is that this initial consultation between patient and team may be the most important initial step towards the successful rehabilitation which subsequently follows. The conference is chaired by the physician responsible for the present and future care of the patients while in the center. It provides a fertile field for the projection of his philosophy; and the physician who is genuinely enthusiastic, optimistic, and interested in the rehabilitation of the stroke patient will call forth the same response from the team. Obviously the many individuals and specific disciplines represented on the team will not work well together unless there is some central direction. Just as the individual therapist must relate to his patient and inspire respect, affection, and a desire to perform well, the physician must relate to the team and inspire them if he expects their results to be consistently successful.

There are four prerequisites which must be fulfilled to make the conference technique successful.

First, prior information concerning the patient's medical problems and disability must be available. This is routine as far as inpatients are concerned because admission to the hospital has been prompted by physician or hospital referral, and in most instances records have been forwarded to the rehabilitation center. Before presentation at the conference, the patient has also undergone the hospital admission workup with history, physical examination, laboratory data, and summation of previous medical information. The data concerning outpatients may be less complete. An attempt to increase this is made by having the patient report to the social service department before conference time and a brief history of the problem is elicited from the patient. Frequently patients also have referring letters from physicians, but some patients come to the center through other patient referral and some through self-referral. If the patient's problem is obscure and it does not seem possible to define it in the time allotted and in the group situation, the patient is given another appointment and undergoes more adequate investigation. Although the possession of this medical information is helpful, it does not exclude the possibility that on some occasions, the referring diagnosis, arrived at through conventional medical investigation, may be proven wrong by an astute diagnostition during such a conference. For instance, patients have been referred as cerebrovascular accidents whose objective findings were atypical enough to stimulate further investigation which established the diagnosis of spinal cord tumor, arterial disease of the spinal cord, a demyelinating disease, and in one instance multiple myeloma.

The second and most important prerequisite is that the patient be informed that he is to be "evaluated" before the entire group in a conference setting. It is a traumatic experience for any patient to appear for evaluation and suddenly find himself before a large audience. Adequate prior preparation for the experience has worked out to be at least 98 per cent successful. There has been only one person who absolutely refused to be seen in this setting, and those few who entered feeling very apprehensive rapidly lost their apprehension once the assessment was underway.

For inpatients this preparation is usually accomplished by the nursing personnel on the rehabilitation ward, under the direction of either the rehabilitation supervisor or the head nurse. This information is imparted to the outpatients during their interview with the social worker prior to the conference. The patients must be told that they are coming into a group situation where they will be sitting before a fairly large size audience, talking with the physician. It should be explained that all individuals present are professional staff members of the team who will be concerned with their care, and the more firsthand knowledge each team member has about their particular disability, the better job may in the long run be done. The patients must be made to feel that the group is here, not for educational purposes, nor for the utilization of patients as guinea pigs, but only because all therapists, etc., are vitally concerned with the care and prognosis of the patient and at least one of these individuals or all collectively may be closely involved in the therapeutic program which is subsequently to be outlined. The patient at this time also become a member of the team.

Unimpeachable group docorum is the third prerequisite. This requires the collective attentiveness, silence, and interest of the *entire* group from the moment the patient walks through the door of the conference room until the patient leaves. There is nothing more distressing or anxiety-creating to the patient when he walks through the door or when he sits before the group than to have team members whispering to each other, talking to each other, or laughing amongst themselves. The first and natural reaction of the patient is to feel that these nonfriendly reactions are related to him, even though the subject matter of the conversation and the cause of the laughter may be quite remote. It should be realized that no matter how large the group, one person who is inattentive, or two people who talk together, or anyone who laughs, all stand out like the proverbial sore thumb. Group tensions therefore must be released and restlessness expended in between patient interviews. The moment the patient walks through the door and during the entire time he is within the room, all members involved in the conference must give undivided and sympathetic attention to the patient, so that in essence, the patient begins to feel that he is not a stranger who is going to be judged by this group tribunal, but that he is actually a member of the team. It may be necessary to repeatedly caution the group about this type of behavior, for carelessness is a common human attribute and personnel does change from time to time.

The last prerequisite is self-evident and charges the physician-in-charge to not only lead the conference, but to make the patient feel as much at ease as possible under the existing circumstances. The approach to this problem again must be varied and depends to a large extent upon the patient, his mental status, his disability, his recent activities, his sense of humor, etc. The exploration towards this assessment may be a cheerful welcoming "Hello" and a comment or question about the weather. If the patient has been brought to the center from another hospital after a prolonged hospitalization, a query may be made concerning his enjoyment of an ambulance ride or change of atmosphere. Attractive items of wearing apparel, especially for female outpatients may be mentioned with a complimentary comment. Many elderly patients enjoy a bit of light exchange concerning their age. No specific guide lines can be laid down to govern this initial exchange but some common ground must be found upon which the physician and the patient can relate to each other in a positive way. The use of pertinent humor is always very helpful towards this goal. Most patients can relate to a bit of appropriate comedy and many patients are actually very good at this themselves. An interesting give and take can occur between patient and physician which not only sets the patient more at ease, but also keeps the whole conference more lively for the other participants as well.

Once the preliminary amenities have been observed, one proceeds to the work at hand. The patient is briefly given a review of the information which the physician has obtained through available sources. The patient is then able to confirm, disagree with, or add to the information which so far has been compiled. Further specific questioning is accomplished at this time to define for the group as clearly as possible the symptomatology and the residual disability which the patient feels subjectively. Although the reason stroke patients are referred to the rehabilitation center is usually quite obvious, in some instances (especially amongst outpatients) it becomes less well defined, and a definite attempt is made to have the patient state in his own words why he has come for help, or how he feels he might be helped. Following the clarification and confirmation of historical data, a gross assessment of the presenting physical disability is made. This gross assessment highlights all visible defects and is sufficient in most instances to determine whether or not the patient should be accepted into the active rehabilitation program. Once acceptance has been accomplished, additional specific investigation is carried out which helps in the specific detailing of the therapeutic program.

The first and most obvious disability noted may be the patient's ability or lack of ability to speak. This information may have been included in referral material, but it becomes much more vivid when actually observed. The written word on the hospital history can never substitute for the actual experience of seeing the patient's reaction or attempted reaction to normal communication. The patient with complete expressive aphasia, but normal cerebration can unwittingly present this utter frustration quite dramatically. The patient with jargon aphasia who feels that he is telling his story quite lucidly and can't quite grasp the look of noncomprehension which is visible in one's eyes and face makes the entire group realize that a major problem in tolerance and understanding lies ahead. During this initial contact, the ability of the patient to comprehend and to obey simple or complex commands can be assessed. This is the most crucial determination to make because patients who are unable to understand and cooperate or obey simple commands will not make successful candidates for rehabilitation.

The objective physical signs of disability are next assessed. It is necessary to determine the side of the body where the current stroke manifests itself. At this time one must also be alert to the fact that some patients have had previous strokes and the so-called present unaffected side may have at one time been the affected one either by a stroke or even by other disabling conditions. Passive and active range of motion of all joints on the affected side must be assessed to see whether or not contractures are present. Contractures are most commonly seen in the shoulder and ankle, and restoration and/or maintenance of this range of motion must be undertaken in the therapeutic program. While one is passively assessing the range of motion of each joint, one also can make a gross assessment of the degree of spasticity which is involved. The most severe spasticity seen is usually in the upper extremity, and on many occasions, even with some return of active motion, it makes this upper extremity nonfunctional. Fortunately, at least in our experience, spasticity in the lower extremity has rarely been the primary cause for inability to ambulate. An assessment of the active motion or strength of the various muscle groups of the upper and lower extremity is next made, as this is necessary in prognosticating the level of achievement which may be successfully obtained. It is important to assess not only the affected side of the body, but the extremities on the unaffected side because if the patient has been bedridden for long periods of time it may also be necessary to provide a strength building program for the so-called normal side. In addition, this side will also have to compensate for the affected side to varying degrees so increased strength for the nonaffected upper and lower extremity can be helpful. In certain instances the patient may have some return of function in the affected extremities, but also have some incoordination which interferes with the fine dexterity. A smaller percentage of patients may also have incoordination on their nonaffected side which is important to demonstrate because this is often a factor in the ability to perform some of the finer techniques of activities of daily living, etc.

Visual defects should be delineated at this time. Homonymous hemianopsia is the most problematical. It is important to point this out to all members of the team, because it can be involved in the rehabilitation process in all areas. The nursing staff needs this information to place the patient properly in his ward unit, so that the available vision can be best utilized. All other groups must realize that the patient should be approached from the side which has vision and that activities and projects should also be initiated from this side. It enhances staff understanding to know that some seemingly uncooperative, recalcitrant patient may only be a patient with a homonymous hemianopsia who has been approached from the wrong side and who is unaware of the various attempts to involve him from his blind side.

The patient is also checked for any deficiencies in sensation on the affected side because many of these patients will be receiving some type of heat to assist in stretching contractures or in eliminating pain. Carelessness can lead to burns.

Having completed the above assessment one can determine whether the patient should be accepted into an active rehabilitation program or rejected.

Criteria for acceptance vary widely depending upon the particular rehabilitation center involved and its philosophy. There are some centers, for instance, who will not accept stroke patients unless they have 15 to 25 per cent return of active motion on the affected side. This means that all patients with complete hemiplegia are rejected even though it can be demonstrated that 15 to 20 per cent of them can be taught to walk successfully independently, and many more can at least become independent in wheelchair activities and independent with minor assistance in activities of daily living. This is certainly better than being bedridden for the rest of one's life. The criteria in this center are fairly simple. The patient must be mentally alert so that he can cooperate and follow simple commands and instructions. It must also be possible to set realistic goals for the patient which will improve not only his own individual place in life, but also make it easier for those who may be involved in his future care. It is also felt that since rejection is so final and the ensuing outlook is so empty, patients who have rated a questionable prognosis should at least be given a limited trial period to see how much progress can be made. All patients are continued in the program as long as they show adequate progress towards realistic goals of independent living, or independent living with minor assistance. A rejection of a patient is made only after careful and due deliberation. The most consistant type of rejection is the outpatient who has had adequate recovery except for the affected upper extremity and who feels rehabilitation techniques can restore a functionless arm. In many instances this is due to the fact that the people who have previously been in charge of the patient's care have not realistically prognosticated his problem and have held out false hope. This often keeps the patient from making the effort to become adequate in all spheres with the remaining nonaffected upper extremity.

After each patient's assessment a brief discussion is allowed and anything which has not been made clear about the patient's story or physical problems is then clarified. Constructive comments from experienced participating therapists may be in order at this time and additional comments from the other therapeutic modalities concerning the prognosis of this patient as it relates to their particular specialty may be sought. When all of the patients have been seen and discussed, a brief intermission is held so that everyone can get up, have a coffee or tea break, etc., and prepare for the remainder of the session.

Upon reconvening from the brief intermission, the business of the team conference continues. X-rays which have been taken since the last meeting are shown to the group and discussed. This visually acquaints the staff with the exact status of a fracture or degree of joint destruction or extensiveness of osteoporosis, etc. The latter is of significance in regard to the stroke patient because one of the major hazards of an active rehabilitation program is the overzealous manipulation of osteoporotic limbs. Prior knowledge of its existence may prevent many iatrogenic fractures. Physicians unfortunately often fail to point out to physical therapists and nurses the degree of osteoporosis which might be present in any particular patient. This omission courts future disaster. Therefore the presentation of patient's x-rays followed by constant verbal reminders of the presence and danger of osteoporosis forewarns all therapists, and projected therapeutic programs are modified accordingly.

A round table discussion involving the entire staff is next conducted. Each member of the staff is called upon for any comments or questions concerning the patients currently in the program. This is the time when therapists bring up specific patients who seem to be making little or no progress in their program in order to find out what progress the patient is making under the other programs involved. At times misunderstandings between staff and patients, or mismatches of temperament and personality may be discovered by such transfer of information. In many instances data provided by the social worker relative to the patient's relationship with his family and home contributes to the understanding of an individual problem. When the last staff member has finished his comments, the conference may proceed to educational matters.

At intervals during the month varied educational exercises are presented. The pathologist assists the group understanding of actual stroke-causing lesions by brain-cutting sessions. Many types of cerebral diseases are demonstrated which can manifest themselves by the stroke syndrome. The staff is able to develop an intricate understanding of the arterial supply to the brain and the various pathological lesions which create the diseases with which they work. A neurologist presents a discussion on interesting cases proposed by the group about whom more information and understanding is desirable. Interesting cases with hand problems are seen by the hand surgeon who joins the conference to discuss the various surgical possibilities which might be employed to improve the situation. Difficult orthopedic problems are also seen and discussed by the orthopedic surgeon who presents his views and recommendations to the staff.

The conference technique when utilized in a positive way can be a most vital factor in ensuring team cooperation and interaction. It provides more understanding of patient and staff problems and serves as a major source of stimulation to all participants.

Chapter VI

ROLE OF THE PHYSICIAN

T HE PHYSICIAN OF today must be prepared to assume a variety of roles in the care of his patients. As a member of the rehabilitation team which includes paramedical personnel, the physician must give effective leadership. All members look to him for guidance, direction, and enlightenment. The stroke patient specifically requires the attention of the physician in two major areas.

GENERAL MEDICAL AREA

When a patient suffers a stroke the family physician is usually called or the patient is taken to a hospital. It may be that the patient has been seen by a physician with this set of symptoms and physical findings, and the first responsibility is that of making an accurate diagnosis. The next is to institute whatever acute therapeutic measures are necessary. Stroke patients may present themselves with a variety of symptom complexes and the acute medical management obviously will differ depending upon each situation. If the patient is comatose it will be necessary to maintain nourishment and hydration by artifical means. It may also be necessary to treat pulmonary infections with antibiotics or airway congestion by suctioning. The patient who is alert and only has minimal to moderate disability may not need such measures. There are certain preventive measures, however, which are unfortunately not universally used today which should be instituted as routine measures at the onset of the stroke. These measures will prevent the common complications which result in many patient-days of morbidity and suffering during rehabilitation.

Contractures

The prevention of contractures in the affected upper and

lower extremities is one of the most important things to accomplish during the initial care of the stroke patient. Too little emphasis has been placed upon this and some 60 per cent of the patients enter our rehabilitation center with severe contractures of the upper extremity. These most commonly involve the shoulder, but the elbow and hand are next in frequency. About 40 per cent of the patients enter with contractures of the lower extremity, usually the ankle, in plantar flexion but also the knee and hip in flexion. A contracture of the upper extremity, if it cannot be reversed, may make it impossible for the patient to achieve total independence in dressing activities as they relate to the upper part of the body. A contracture of the lower extremity of equal severity may prevent the patient from ever walking again. These contractures are very painful to stretch,

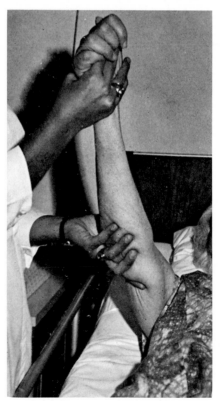

FIGURE 1. Nurse putting affected upper extremity through passive range of motion. Shoulder flexion phase is illustrated.

and many patients will not tolerate the procedure. Surgical intervention may become necessary.

The simplest thing, therefore, is to prevent them. This can be accomplished by performing adequate passive range of motion of all joints of the affected and even unaffected extremities if the patient is not moving the latter himself. This entails maneuvering each joint through each of its range of motion capabilities for ten repetitions at least six times a day. This procedure can be taught to nurses of all levels of training, to more dependable nurses aides, to family members, and even to the patient himself when he becomes alert. However, this preventive procedure is never done unless the physician takes the initiative, recognizes its need, and includes it in the routine written orders (see Fig. 1).

In addition to passive range of motion it is also necessary to properly position the affected upper and lower extremities when the patient is in bed, when sitting in a chair, and when in a standing position. During the time the patient is in bed, the upper extremity should be placed to the side of the body in an abducted position with the hand on a pillow, so that the wrist is above the elbow and the elbow is above the shoulder (see Fig. 2). A soft roll is placed in the hand to prevent flexion deformity of the fingers if necessary. The patient should be well down in the bed so that the foot is held at a right angle against the footboard in a neutral position and with the heel off the mattress in a trough between the end of the mattress and the footboard (see Fig. 3). The leg is maintained in the neutral position by sand bags or a trochanter roll (see Chap. VII, Fig. 26 and 27).

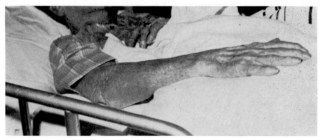

FIGURE 2.   Affected upper extremity positioned on pillows when patient is supine in bed.

In the sitting position the upper extremity should again be protected by placing it on a pillow or armboard fastened to the arm of the wheelchair (see Figs. 4-6). This is positioned to

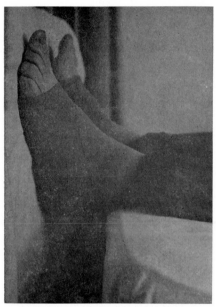

FIGURE 3. Lower extremity positioned in neutral against footboard. Heel is free from pressure as it lies in trough between footboard and mattress.

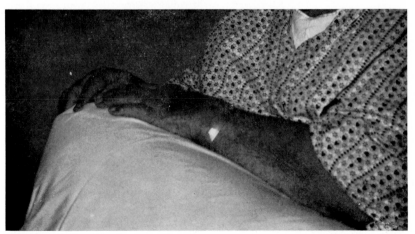

FIGURE 4. Paralyzed or weakened upper extremity positioned on pillows when sitting in chair.

maintain some degree of abduction of the shoulder and elevation of the wrist. A real spastic upper extremity may be put in a right angle outrigger on the wheelchair with straps and slings, so that the paralyzed upper extremity will be held in even greater abduction and the wrist and elbow are slightly elevated to prevent contracture formation and edema (see Figs. 7 and 8). The

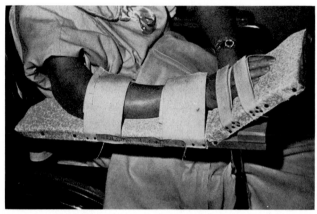

FIGURE 5.   Arm board designed to fit on wheelchair arm to hold affected upper extremity in desired position. Velcro straps provide the necessary confinement.

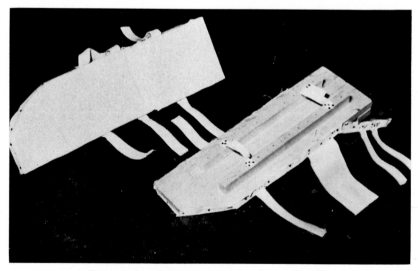

FIGURE 6.   Component parts of arm board.

lower extremity can be properly positioned by using an elevated leg rest and can be maintained in the proper neutral position by a Velcro strap around the calf (see Figs. 9 and 10).

In the standing position, the patient with a flaccid upper extremity should wear a sling to maintain the integrity of the shoulder and prevent edema of the hands (see Figs. 11-13). The lower extremity should be properly braced with temporary dorsiflexor assists (see Figs. 14-16).

As needed, splinting for the hand and wrist using simple hand rolls, boards with hand rolls or actual static splints constructed from different commercial materials should be used. Prefabricated splints are also available commercially for this use (see Figs. 17-21).

A movie entitled "The Stroke Patient—Parts I, II, III, and IV" is available from the Massachusetts Heart Association and demon-

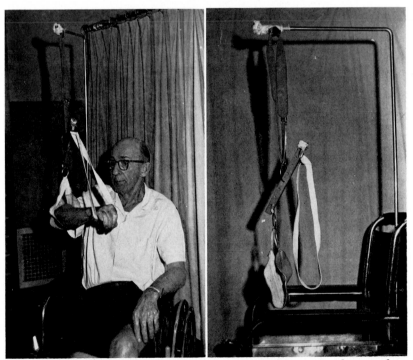

FIGURE 7. A spastic upper extremity is positioned by using slings and an outrigger attached to the wheelchair.

FIGURE 8. Component parts of outrigger attachment.

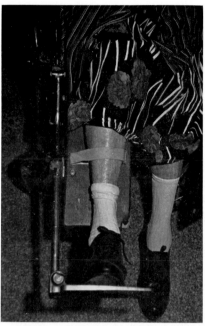

FIGURE 9.   Lower extremity positioned on elevated leg rest and held by Velcro strap.

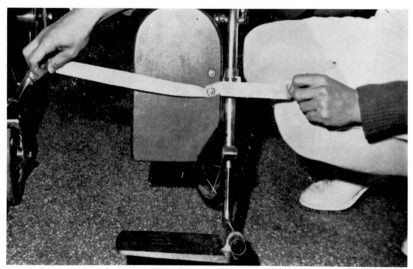

FIGURE 10.   Velcro strap is attached to screw on leg rest.

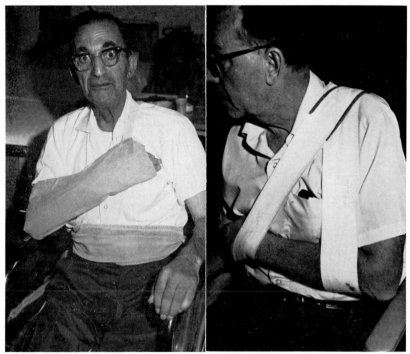

FIGURE 11. One type of arm sling used to support affected shoulder and prevent edema of hand. It is inexpensive, washable, and can be easily put on and taken off by patient himself. Only used for flaccid extremity in standing position.

FIGURE 12. A second type of arm sling currently being studied. Purposes and application are the same as those in FIGURE 11.

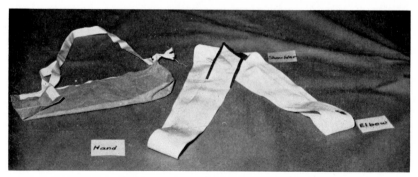

FIGURE 13. Component parts of arm slings.

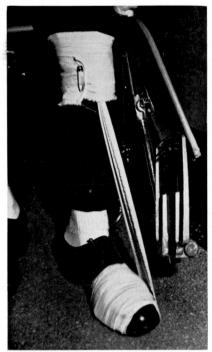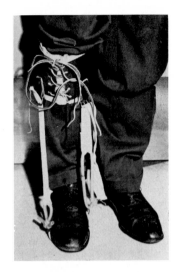

Figure 14.   An Ace bandage temporary assist provides dorsiflexion and eversion in a foot with little spasticity.

Figure 15.   Temporary assist providing more tensil strength. It is used for more spastic feet. It requires insertion of wire through medial and lateral edge of shoe sole.

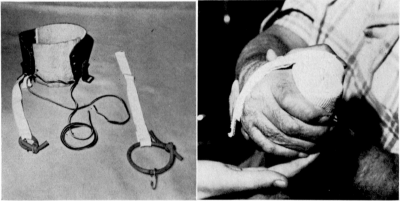

Figure 16.   Component parts of temporary assist. It requires leather cuff lined with foam rubber, lacing, webbing, rubber tubing, and wire.

Figure 17.   Hand roll held in place by Velcro strap. It prevents severe finger flexion.

strates the methods of patient evaluation as well as how to do range of motion, proper positioning, and splinting. A pamphlet "Strike Back at Stroke," with drawings of range of motion techniques is available from the chronic illness section of the Department of Health, Education, and Welfare in Washington, D. C.

The extreme necessity to institute these preventive measures

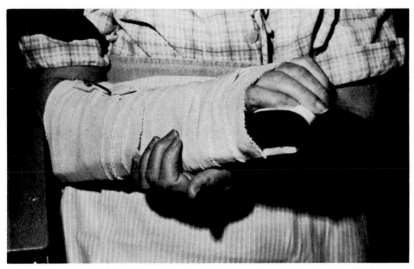

FIGURE 18. Arm board with felt padding held in place by an Ace bandage. This prevents flexion deformity of wrist and hand.

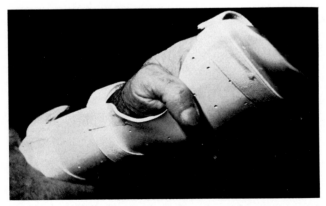

FIGURE 19. A Royalite splint held in place by Velcro straps. Material is heated in an oven and shaped over a plaster mold because it is too hot to apply directly to the skin.

for the joints cannot be stressed enough because many of the rehabilitation procedures required later on are directed towards

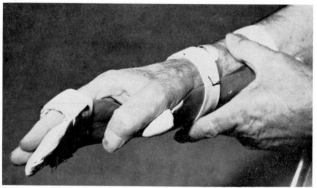

FIGURE 20. Fiberglass splint is more complicated to make but produces most durable, lightweight, easily cleanable splint. Fabrication requires first a negative plaster mold of the hand, then a positive mold made from Duroc. Fiberglass is then placed over the mold which has been rubbed in orthofree and coated with orthobond A and B mixed 4 parts to 1 respectively. More mixture is applied and another layer of fiberglass. It is allowed to dry and then is heated in an oven at 180 degrees for 30 minutes. It must be trimmed, sanded, and have orthofree removed with a knife. Finally another coat of mixture is applied inside and out and it is again placed in the oven for 30 minutes at 180 degrees. Newer splinting materials include Prenyl, Orthoplast and Bio-plastic all three of which can be heated in warm water and molded to shape.

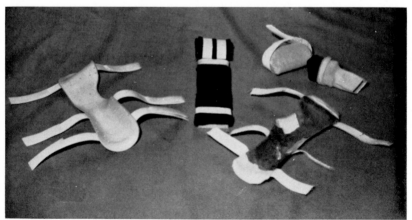

FIGURE 21. The assorted splints as they appear when not in use.

reversing contractures which should not have happened in the first place. Maintenance of adequate range of motion also insures the patient's being able to use this extremity at a later date should active useful function return.

Bed Sores

The prevention of bedsores is admittedly not exclusively a problem of stroke patients. This problem is known only too well to all physicians and nurses who care for all types of bed patients. However it is especially depressing and distressing for the stroke patient who has so many other disabilities, to be held back in his progress by large deep decubiti which often take months and months to heal. In addition to the morbidity imposed, the hospital stay is prolonged and the cost of care increased. The best way to prevent this problem is to recognize that these patients should be mobilized from the bed as soon as they achieve some degree of mental alertness. However, the act of taking the patient out of bed and placing him in a chair for hours does not entirely prevent this problem. The patient must also be moved periodically or taught to move himself periodically to alternate pressure points. The skin should be watched constantly for any reddened areas and proper attention given to

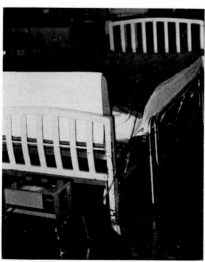

Figure 22. Alternating pulsating air mattress.

such areas immediately. Should the patient have to stay in bed because of justifiable reasons, frequent turning, alternating pulsating mattresses, total flotation mattresses, Stryker frames, use of sheepskin, Circ-o-lectric beds as well as impeccable hygiene, etc., must all be considered (see Figures 22-24).

As stated above about contractures, the best treatment for decubiti is total prevention. The physician must again therefore take the initiative to see that one or all of the above measures are being employed to prevent the occurrence of bedsores on his patient. He should check the patient's potential trouble spots daily himself to see that all proper precautions are being faithfully taken.

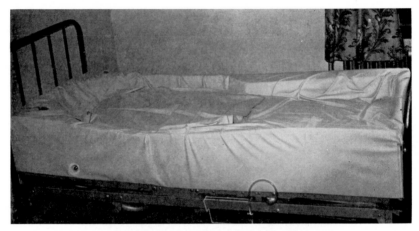

FIGURE 23.   Flotation mattress.

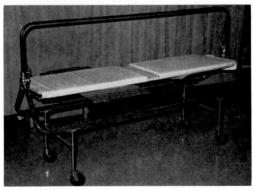

FIGURE 24.   Stryker frame.

Bladder Volume

Unfortunately it has become almost traditional for the doctor to insert, or have inserted a catheter into the urinary bladder should the patient show any degree of incontinence. In fact many patients are catheterized before they have a chance to qualify. With certain types of patients, such as the comatose person who is unable to cooperate, this may be justified. However, making this decision should entail more than routinely saying, "Put the patient on constant drainage."

Catheterization is not a benign procedure. A number of things happen when a catheter is placed in the bladder. Most common is the development of bladder infections. These are usually easily managed at a later date by using appropriate antibiotics. They might have been suppressed by the concomitant use of moderate doses of medication such as Gantrisin® or Mandelamine®, coupled with adequate fluid intake and sometimes cranberry juice. However the major problem by far is the subsequent loss of bladder volume. This is actually caused by contractures of the muscles of the bladder wall which occur when a catheter is left in place for long periods of time keeping the bladder itself empty. Preventing normal filling of the bladder to its limit in effect decreases its range of motion and results in decreased capacity. This can be prevented by the use of tidal drainage, by the use of modified duke's drainage (where the Y tube is maintained about four to six inches above the pubis and the bladder has to fill and build up some intervesicular pressure in order to push the urine up over the gradient and into the bottle), or by intermittently clamping the catheter off for periods of time.

However, many of these patients are alert and do not require catheters in the first place. The nurses must spend some time studying the patients' voiding patterns and put them on the toilet at routine intervals. In this way most of these patients will void and keep dry. It is routine in our rehabilitation center for all catheters to be removed from patients upon admission, and it is the rare and unusual patient who cannot be controlled as far as voiding is concerned. The patients who create the most difficulty are those who have previously had catheters and who now have contracted bladders holding small amounts of urine.

They must go to the bathroom very frequently until this can be improved and this often retards the rehabilitation process. Voiding at night can be controlled by bedpanning at regular intervals until a commode or regular toilet can be safely used. The basic principle is to allow the patient to void into a receptacle prior to his need to void wherever he may be. It is very frustrating to therapists who must work with such patients because a great deal of therapy time is utilized by going to and from the bathroom. A bladder of normal volume, therefore, is a great asset to the stroke patient who wishes to return home and to the community. The doctor must insist upon better bladder care and management and not give in quite so easily to the nurse's request to catheterize the patient because this may make her task simpler.

Dehydration

It may seem odd that this type of problem should be discussed. It is common knowledge that all general hospitals through their nursing staffs have routines to provide receptacles and cups on every patient's bedside table, and the water is changed two or three times a day. A doctor probably never notices how many times a full pitcher of water is picked up and exchanged for another each day, and in many instances the patient has received little or no fluid intake. A dehydrated patient is often lethargic and prostrate and falsely gives the impression that he has no rehabilitation potential. A number of patients have entered our rehabilitation center presenting this wilted, weakened appearance. Following a week of concentrated attention to improving their state of hydration, they become alert, active, and excellent candidates for the program. Therefore the physician should see to it that the patient gets adequate fluid intake during his acute illness in the general hospital or at home. This will help the patient present himself in a better light, project a more hopeful image, and possibly give the physician more assurance that he is a candidate for rehabilitation.

Weakness of Disuse

In certain patients, especially those in the geriatric group, extended periods of time in bed are detrimental. The physiological problems created by prolonged bed rest are well known. However, little attention seems to be paid to the marked degree of physical disability which can be created in an older person by unjustified bed rest. The final result is a patient who not only has a paralyzed or weak side caused by the stroke, but who also develops very weak nonaffected extremities and back muscles. Actual atrophy and flabbiness may occur. This means that the patient has to be physically rehabilitated on both the affected and nonaffected sides and significantly increases the magnitude and the cost of the job at hand. This is a major reason for the stroke patient to be mobilized out of the bed and allowed to participate in physical activities as soon as possible. The alert patient with a thrombus or an embolus, could be out of bed within forty-eight hours. The patient with a cerebral hemorrhage or subarachnoid hemorrhage should be mobilized as soon as his medical situation warrants.

Fecal Impactions

About 30 per cent of the patients referred to this center from general hospitals need disimpaction upon admission. It is evident that the routine order for milk of magnesia or mineral oil is not enough to ensure regularity in many people. Physical inactivity, change of diet, decreased fluid intake, bedpan embarrassment, etc., combine to make this routine daily occurrence a major problem in medical management. Early mobility, proper diet, adequate fluid intake, judicious use of a variety of cathartics, stool softeners, suppositories, but above all, privacy for the patient in the act of defecation should be provided. The patient's experience will depend directly upon the doctor's interest in, understanding of, and active involvement in the bowel program.

SPECIFIC AREAS

All physicians who are responsible for the care of stroke patients should certainly take the responsibility for the direction and supervision of the situations discussed above. Physicians who are also to be involved in the progressive rehabilitation of these patients to their maximum level of independence must be prepared to accomplish what is discussed below.

Evaluation

If the rehabilitation process is to be meaningful and is to proceed in a precise manner, a gross evaluation of the patient's actual disability must be made. During examination, each extremity is assessed for the presence of voluntary active muscle power. The active muscle groups are recorded and their relative strength tested. Presence of spasticity and degree of severity are noted. Passive range of joint mobility is next checked and any deficiencies listed. Contractures in particular are sought and demonstrated. A finger-nose test and rapid alternating movements is done to highlight the presence of incoordination. It is also well to examine the nonaffected extremity for incoordination because at times this is involved and complicates the rehabilitation process. It is very important to confirm the presence of homonymous hemianopsia as the treatment plan in all areas will need modification to circumvent the problems associated with this loss. Any other visual problems should be documented and the patient's reliance upon glasses stressed. Deficits in cutaneous sensation must be outlined especially if heat is to be used as part of the treatment. The general physical condition and state of hydration should be assessed, and if x-rays are available and osteoporosis is evident, this is the opportune time to caution the therapists.

Once the assets and liabilities have been tabulated, one uses this information to proceed to the next specific step.

Setting of Goals

The goals for each patient must be tailor-made for his problems. They should be preventive, progressive, understandable, and above all, attainable. In a paralyzed extremity, the goal is to maintain range of motion of all joints and prevent contracture formation. When slight weak motion has returned, the goal is to foster and assist this strength to increase. If the extremity has a fair amount of return of power, the aim is to make it stronger. If a contracture is present, the goal is to stretch it. If there is pain in any area, the goal is to relieve it. When a patient has been bedridden for a long period of time, the goal is to accustom him to the upright position in preparation for standing. If the patient has severe spasticity, the goal is to relieve this as much as possible. For the incoordinated extremity the goal is to produce a patient who is as independent in activities of daily living and ambulation as possible. Additional goals may be set depending upon the patient's performance. The creation of these goals provides the foundation material for the third specific step.

Writing of Orders

To start the patient actively participating in the program, written orders outlining the treatment plan should be supplied to the various departments for the guidance of the therapists. Orders written for the physical therapy department, for example, may be as follows: If the patient has a painful shoulder, some type of heat modality such as a hot pack might be ordered before exercise. If a contracture is present, an order to use passive and active stretch should be considered. The person who continues to have a paralyzed extremity may require an order to maintain the range of motion of all joints by passive exercise. If the extremity is very weak, assistive exercises may be used. As the extremity becomes stronger, active exercises should be instituted, and as the extremity becomes even stronger, progressive resistive exercises will be appropriate. Should it be necessary to accustom the patient to the upright position, tilt table time should be ordered. As soon as proficiency is achieved on the tilt table, the patient should progress to standing and walking in the parallel bars, next to using a walking aid outside of the parallel bars, and finally ambulation without a walking aid, if possible. Concurrently orders written for occupational therapy would also include maintaining range of motion of a paralyzed upper extremity, increasing the strength of a weak upper extremity, increasing the strength and dexterity of the nonaffective upper extremity (especially if it is the nondominant one), increasing the patient's overall physical endurance, increasing the endurance for standing when the ability has been achieved, checking out the activities of daily living to see whether any devices may be necessary, and with women, checking them out in household activities. The occupational therapist may then choose from a number of craft modalities to bring about the desired results.

The patient is reevaluated periodically for progress, and any changes in therapy may be suggested as needed. At the proper time the nursing staff also becomes involved in supervision and instruction of transfer techniques, dressing, bathing, and feeding activities; and it helps provide endurance in ambulation. The patient's family is referred to the Social Service Department upon admission so that social problems if present may receive immediate attention. The social worker functions as a very active member of the team, not just a vehicle of patient disposition. Speech evaluation and therapy should be ordered for the patient who has any difficulty in communication. This department should also be requested to test the hearing of any patient that the physician feels may have a deficiency in this area. Lack of attention or response is often due to a defect in hearing.

Miscellaneous

There are other specific responsibilities which the physician must accept while caring for his stroke patient. It is his responsibility to provide confidence, reassurance, and optimism for his patient. He must enlighten the family concerning the rehabilitation process and assist them with their anxieties. It is important to demonstrate to the patient that one understands his frustration and fears but that he will improve and make progress if motivated. Far too many physicians still tell the family that there is no hope, that there is nothing positive to be done, that the patient should be put in a nursing home and that is it. By taking the active role portrayed above, the physician will see for himself that there is a new dimension in the current care of the stroke patient.

It is unfortunate to note that most paramedical personnel are much more advanced in the knowledge of stroke patient treatment plans than are physicians and they are capable of furnishing excellent service. Yet they still look to the physician for guidance and the physician must take the leadership in the care and management of his stroke patients as well as all his other patients. If the patient deserves the best medical care available at this time, and if the medical profession is to be respected by paramedical personnel, and if all of these professional services are to be utilized in an organized manner, the physician must be the captain of and set the theme for the team.

Chapter VII

ROLE OF THE NURSE

THE NURSE IS A key member of the team. Her position is unique because she works in a department which gives twenty-four-hour service, seven days a week. The nurse therefore assumes a major responsibility for the stroke patient's care as she is in contact with the patient for more hours of the day than the other disciplines.

The aim is to promote a nursing program for each patient which is in accordance with his own capacity and physical ability. This is accomplished through the attainment of small goals which eventually amalgamate into larger ones.

A successful nursing program depends on a staff thoroughly oriented to its scope and consistent in its approach to and awareness of each patient's goals. Although it is demanding to orient an entire staff to the concepts and skills required in a rehabilitation program, attainment of such promotes a more cohesive, functional program for the patient. The everyday contact of the staff with the patient and with one another is crucial because it is not one member of the nursing staff but many who are providing care throughout the day. Consistency in approach is the key to this type of program if the person with a hemiplegia is to progress to his maximum independence with a minimum of confusion and frustration. Because the nurse's role is not the traditional one of "doing" for the patient, but one of assisting him in doing things for himself, *it is reflected in all her activities with him.* The nurse becomes a teacher and continually evaluates his abilities by questioning.

1. What is he doing?
2. What is he unable to do?
3. What methods can be utilized to help him to achieve his potential?

4. What is being done for him that he can do himself?

5. Are all staff members equally aware of his problems and using the same method of instruction?

This silent self-interrogation begins at the time of admission when the initial nursing evaluation is done.

In order to develop a nursing plan one must know the following:

1. Can the patient communicate?

2. What are his abilities in self-care?

3. Is he continent? Has he been on a catheter or a type of modified tidal drainage?

4. Does he have difficulty with constipation, diarrhea, or impaction?

5. What is the condition of his skin?

6. Has he been out of bed? For how long?

7. Is he able to maneuver his wheelchair?

TABLE III
INITIAL NURSING EVALUATION FORM

NAME

DIAGNOSIS

Aphasia	*Visual Impairment*
Expressive	Hemianopsia
Receptive	Blind
	Visual loss
Concomitant factors	
Memory loss	*Bowel*
Short Attention Span	Impacted
Confused	Constipation
Unable to follow verbal command	Diarrhea
Poor judgment	Laxatives
Bladder	*Mouth*
Catheter	
Continent	*Length of Time*
Incontinent	
	Eating
Skin	
Dry	*Transfer*
Dehydrated	
Reddened areas	*Wheelchair mobility*
Pressure areas	
Out of bed daily?	
Self-care	
Hygiene	
Dressing	
Nursing goals	

8. Is he able to transfer independently, with assistance, or is he dependent?

9. Does he have a visual or hearing defect?

10. Does he have a sensory loss?

11. Does he present any concomitant phenomena such as memory loss, short attention span, inability to concentrate, confusion, poor judgment?

Assets and liabilities are balanced and the nursing plan takes shape.

A nursing evaluation form is completed during the first twenty-four to forty-eight hours of admission (see Table III). An ADL (activities of daily living) card is filled out and placed in the file. The purpose of such a card is to provide information in one central place where all staff may find it. The card is primarily a checklist with some space for other specific information. It assists the nursing staff and other members of the rehabilitation team in providing more meaningful care (see Table IV).

TABLE IV
ADL CARD

NAME   DIAGNOSIS

Washes in	*Dressing*	*Ambulation*	*Vision*
wheelchair	underpants	walks	good
bathroom	shorts	independent	impaired
bed	pedal pushers	supervision with	glasses
tub	trousers	cane	hemianopsia
	bra	regular	
Washes	shirt	4-pronged	*Hearing*
face	blouse	crutches	good
neck	socks	regular	loss
arms	shoes	loftstrand	aid
trunk		walker	
perineum	brace		*Aphasia*
legs	splint	*Restraint*	expressive
back	sling	wheelchair	receptive
	ace bandage	bed	both
Grooming			
hair	*Fasteners*	*Transfer*	
teeth	zippers		
dentures	buttons	*Eating*	
nails	shoelace	independent	
makeup	shoe zippers	assist	
shave	elastic laces	adaptive equip.	
		plate guard	
		other	

SCALE: 1 = independent, 2 = supervision, 3 = assistance.

PREVENTION OF SUPERIMPOSED DEFORMITIES

Contracture prevention is basic to any rehabilitation program. Since the nurse is one of the first disciplines to manage the patient her conscientious effort to prevent such complications can influence the length and cost of hospitalization. Of primary importance is the maintenance of joint mobility. Restriction in joint mobility can hinder his ability in such things as self-care, eating, ambulation, and transfer activities. Normal joint mobility may be maintained by passive range of motion, proper positioning, and proper splinting.

Range of Motion

Range of motion can be defined as the extent of expected normal movement in a given joint. It is also the technique of placing a joint or joints through the normal range of motion. This procedure not only is a means of maintaining mobile joints, but it prevents pain resulting from tight muscles and ligaments. Range of motion, as a nursing measure, is employed to *maintain* mobility which is present. Its importance in nursing care must be recognized and it must be actually carried out in a planned program. Many nurses feel that range of motion, as a nursing procedure, is not necessary when the patient is participating in a physical therapy program. This is not correct when one recognizes the difference in the primary purpose of each of these disciplines as they relate to the performance of range of motion. Emphasis is placed on treating the affected extremities, but the unaffected extremities may also at times need to be included. The patient, when alert, can be instructed to do this himself and should be encouraged to actively participate (see Chap. VIII, Fig. 66).

When placing a person's joints through passive range of motion the following rules apply:

1. Position the patient in proper body alignment and make him as comfortable as possible.

2. Encourage him to do as much of the motion as he is able while keeping your hands in a position of support.

3. Support the extremity at the joints.

4. Physical contact should be gentle (do not grasp with

fingers but hold in the palms of hands).

5. Do not go beyond the point of pain.

6. Movements should be gentle, slow and rhythmic, pausing at the completion of each movement.

Proper Positioning

The upper extremity frequently develops a painful shoulder, limited in motion. This can inhibit the ability to do daily tasks such as dress the upper part of the body, comb and brush the hair, fasten a bra, etc.

When in bed the affected upper extremity is at times placed in the so-called stop position with the shoulder abducted and externally rotated. The hand can be placed under the pillow (see Fig. 25). During other periods it may be propped on pillows so that the shoulder is abducted and the hand elevated above the elbow and the elbow above the shoulder (see Chap. IV, Fig. 2). The upper extremity may also be positioned with the shoulder in 90 degrees of abduction, the elbow extended and partially supinated. Sandbags placed in apposition with

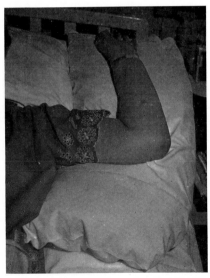

FIGURE 25. Affected upper extremity placed in "stop" position when patient lies supine in bed.

the arm maintain its position. The stop position or pillow support can also be used in the prone position.

If the patient is in a chair, the affected upper extremity is positioned in a similar way by using pillows, by constructing a suitable armrest, or in the case of very spastic arms, by attaching a right angle outrigger with slings and springs to the chair. The basic principle is to prevent flexion deformities, adduction, subluxation of the shoulder, and peripheral edema (see Chap. VI, Figs. 4-8).

While in a standing position, flaccid upper extremities only are placed in a sling. This helps maintain the integrity of the shoulder but must not be used injudiciously (see Chap. VI, Figs. 11-13).

The lower extremity must also be protected. During the time the patient is in bed the foot is placed against a footboard to prevent plantar flexion and shortening of the Achilles tendon (see Chap. VI, Fig. 3). The leg is kept in neutral position by using either sandbags or a trochanter roll (see Figs. 26 and 27). This is done to prevent external rotation of the hip which later is an impediment to the achievement of a good gait pattern. Pillows should never be placed under the knee because this predisposes to flexion contractures of this joint.

When in a wheelchair the leg rests should be adjusted to the

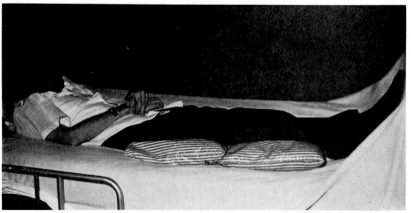

FIGURE 26.   Sandbags placed along the lateral side of affected lower extremity prevent external rotation of the hip.

proper length. Since paralyzed and very weak lower extremities frequently become edematous, the leg rest is usually elevated and the foot maintained in neutral position by a small Velcro strap fastened to the wheelchair by a screw. The strap fits snugly around the lower leg (see Chap. VI, Figs. 9 and 10). The strap fits snugly around the lower leg (see Chap. VI, Figs. 9 and 10).

In the standing position, a posterior splint held in place by

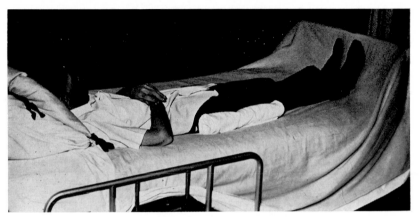

FIGURE 27. A trochanter roll provides another method of preventing external rotation of the affected hip.

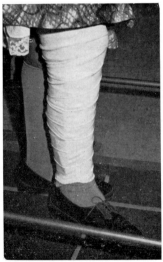

FIGURE 28. Posterior splint held in place with Ace bandage.

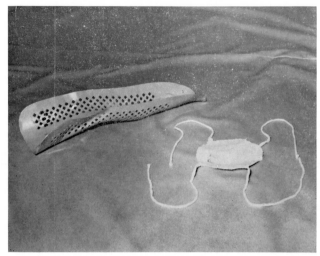

FIGURE 29. Component parts of posterior splint. The knee cap provides additional support by preventing knee flexion.

an ace bandage and kneecap strap is used to give stability to a severely weakened leg (see Figs. 28 and 29). Dorsiflexion at the ankle is maintained by temporary assists. If the foot is not too spastic, an ace bandage assist is applied, otherwise a stronger assist made of leather, foam rubber, rubber tubing, webbing, and wire is fabricated for the patient's use (see Chap. VI, Figs. 14-16).

Although most of the above materials and pieces of small equipment are initiated by the physical therapy department, the nurse must be familiar with all as she will be providing auxillary ambulation or wheelchair supervision during the hours the patient is on the ward.

Proper Splinting

The third requirement for contracture prevention is the use of certain simple static splints which are sometimes used at night as well as throughout the day. These are not fabricated by the nurse but she must know how to apply them properly. She must also be knowledgeable about the application of short- and long-leg braces (see Figs. 30-33).

No one of the three methods discussed above will be com-

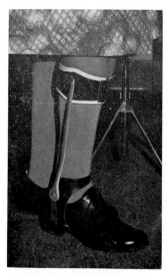
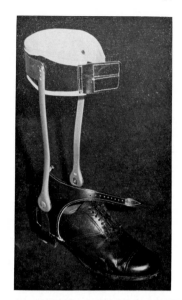

FIGURE 30. Short-leg brace on patient.

FIGURE 31. Short-leg brace with below knee cuff, Klenzak ankle and T strap attached to shoe.

pletely effective alone. A daily routine which includes all must be maintained for the best results.

SKIN CARE

The need for meticulous skin care is especially recognized by the nurse. It is much easier to prevent skin breakdown than to institute and carry through a treatment program. Once the integrity of the skin has been disturbed, delay in physical restoration, frustration, and extra financial burden has been added to both the patient and his family. A decubitus ulcer can prolong hospitalization three months or more. Through the practice of simple measures the nurse can in most instances prevent skin breakdown. These measures are as follows:

1. Daily inspection of the skin for reddened areas.
2. At the first sign of redness find cause of pressure.
3. Remove or alleviate the cause.
4. Massage reddened areas.

Certain areas of the body are more susceptible to pressure from the constant weight of the body. These areas occur over

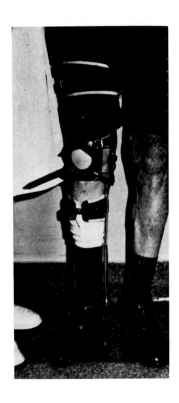
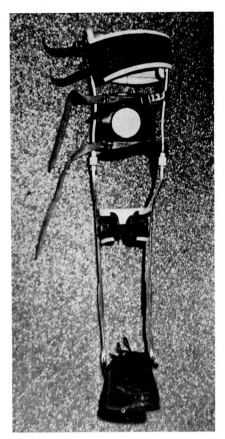

FIGURE 32.   Long-leg brace on patient.

FIGURE 33.   Long-leg brace with thigh and below-knee cuffs, knee support, drop locks, and Klenzak ankle attached to shoe.

the bony prominences such as the sacrum, kneecap, scapula, ankle, heel, and trochanter.

Pressure is alleviated by changing position frequently. The patient is taught to change his position every ten to fifteen minutes when he is sitting in his wheelchair. If he is able, he is encouraged to stand frequently. For those who need assistance, one of the staff is assigned to assist in this task. When in bed, the position of the patient is changed from side to back every two to four hours during the night and/or whenever it is necessary for him to be in bed. Prone lying is advantageous if he is able to tolerate it. It is wise to keep in mind that the patient probably will not like this procedure at first. There is always an element of fear. He will need to have confidence in the person who turns him and he should not be left on his abdomen longer than ten minutes for the first few times. He should not be left alone until he becomes accustomed to it.

The skin can be injured by scraping, rubbing, and/or striking, as well as by remaining in the same position too long. Scraping, rubbing, and/or striking can occur during dressing and transfer activities. A scraped ankle is frequently due to one of the following: striking it against the footpedal during transfer, dressing the lower extremity, friction of the straps used when exercising on the leg press; friction from rolling on the mat in physical therapy or mattress while in bed; or a leg brace which does not fit properly. Assists and splints used to prevent or correct contractures must be watched closely for underlying pressure areas and/or irritation.

If there is a sensory loss on the affected side, the skin becomes even more prone to irritations. The automatic response of withdrawal to discomfort has been lost. Because of this, the patient is taught to be extremely cautious with his affected side. Frequently his arm may become bruised or lacerated from striking it against the arm of the wheelchair or furniture such as the corners of tables. He must also avoid the possibility of burns. Radiators and exposed pipes should be covered, and the temperature of bath water carefully controlled.

Moisture causes irritation and discomfort. For this reason the skin must be dried thoroughly after washing, particularly where skin surfaces touch skin, such as the axilla, perineum, under the breasts, or skin folds. These areas are not open to the air and inadequate drying may lead to problems. The use of absorbent materials is helpful.

Urine on the skin also causes irritation and discomfort if in prolonged contact. Because of this, if the patient is incontinent, dribbles, or unavoidably has an accident, he is washed carefully with warm soapy water and dried thoroughly.

BOWEL AND BLADDER

The demoralization associated with incontinency can be a

deterrent not only to the patient's active participation in portions of his rehabilitation program but also in his desire to socialize and interrelate with others. It is embarrassing for him not to be able to control his bowels and bladder. The fear that he might have a bowel movement or void while in physical therapy, occupational therapy, or during some social activity causes him to withdraw and avoid contact with others. For this reason a bowel and bladder program is instituted upon admission.

The goals of the bowel program are to achieve control of involuntary evacuations, promote regularity, prevent constipation and impaction, prevent skin irritation, and minimize emotional stress. The patient's cooperation must be sought. The success of the program depends upon his willingness to put forth effort and the nursing staff's understanding of the program. Complications such as memory loss, mental confusion, and receptive aphasia can create difficulties but these can usually be overcome with perseverance.

To institute such a program, the nursing staff must be well oriented and understand their responsibilities to the patient. For example, if a suppository is inserted, the nursing personnel must be available to toilet him at the designated time. Faithfulness in maintaining adequate records is paramount. Not only is it necessary to record whether the patient has had a bowel movement, but also the consistency of the stool, the amount, and color should be noted. A history of previous habits is solicited.

Has he had difficulty with constipation? Has he been in the habit of taking laxatives? What has his normal schedule been for evacuation—daily, every other day, etc.? A digital examination is done to rule out the possibility of impaction. If he should be impacted, a cleansing enema and disimpaction is ordered since the bowel should be clear before beginning the program.

A balanced diet with no in-between meals and a fluid intake of at least 1,500 cc (2,000 to 3,000 cc is preferable) is begun. An accurate record of fluid intake and output is kept. Gas-forming foods and foods causing diarrhea or constipation are discouraged, while foods having bulk are encouraged. It is routine for some to have a glass of prune juice daily at breakfast time.

Regularity is also important. Most patients usually choose right after breakfast, although the time may be optional. If at all possible, his usual schedule should be observed. This can be extremely difficult for the nursing staff if there is a shortage of personnel.

Activity is another factor and as much physical activity as possible within his ability, whether it be transfer, wheelchair, ambulation activities, or exercise in therapy should be encouraged. Above all, however, is the need to provide privacy for this personal act. The preservation of human dignity will do more good than many of the other factors.

It is important to realize that incontinency is not always due to a neurologic impairment. Many times urinary incontinency is accepted as inevitable because a person is old or ill. Assessment of each individual person to find the cause of his incontinency is thus neglected. Observation by the nursing personnel becomes extremely important in assisting the physician's assessment. In many instances the patient is incontinent because there is no nurse there to toilet him when he has the urge to void. For this reason stress must be placed upon the importance of answering his call quickly and cheerfully. The toileting schedule should be based on his needs rather than on a routine designed for nursing expediency only. Incontinency can also be due to urologic disorders which are apart from the cerebral vascular accident and once correctly diagnosed are in many instances treatable.

The objectives of a bladder program are as follows:
1. Provide a voiding pattern.
2. Prevent incontinency.
3. Maintain bladder tone.
4. Prevent skin irritation and breakdown.
5. Alleviate emotional stress.

The bladder program can be successful with patience and perseverance. First, the patient's voiding pattern is checked to see whether it is every two hours, three hours, or four hours. Since it is a twenty-four-hour program, each shift of nurses has its responsibility in carrying out the program. Once the rhythm of the pattern has been noted, it is a matter of being present at the correct time to toilet him. If there are toilet facilities available, these are always used in preference to the bedpan since it produces a more normal position for voiding. For those who void at short intervals, the nurse begins to encourage them to hold their urine a bit longer each time until the interval approaches normality.

In the rare instance in which an indwelling catheter must be used, it must be connected to an irrigation apparatus which helps to maintain the tone of his bladder.

This is maintained by inserting a Y tube in the tubing and taping it to the pole approximately four inches above the level of the bladder. The height of the loop is ordered by the physician (see Fig. 34). During the time he is out of bed his catheter is clamped for two hours and then released for twenty minutes. The patient is encouraged to assume this responsibility if he is able. A person having a retention catheter is encouraged to drink four glasses of cranberry juice daily and often may be covered with a suppressive dose of Mandelamine.® This helps to keep the urine acid.

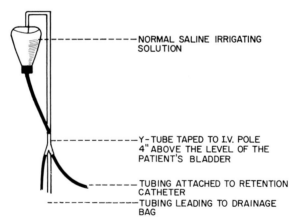

NORMAL SALINE IRRIGATING SOLUTION

Y-TUBE TAPED TO I.V. POLE 4" ABOVE THE LEVEL OF THE PATIENT'S BLADDER

TUBING ATTACHED TO RETENTION CATHETER

TUBING LEADING TO DRAINAGE BAG

FIGURE 34. Diagram of urinary drainage and irrigation system. The Y tube is attached to the pole about 4 to 6 inches above pubic level when the patient is in bed to maintain bladder tone.

SELF-CARE ACTIVITIES

It is important to keep several things in mind when beginning to work with a person in self-care activities. First, the nurse is responsible for encouraging him to do all functional activities such as washing, dressing, eating, transferring, and pushing his wheelchair, as a part of the daily nursing unit routine. Second, the nurse must be aware of the limiting factors which might prevent or limit the performance of these activities. Two major deterrents are severe brain damage and severe loss of physical function. The program must be set up so that too much will not be expected of him.

Disturbances in memory are particularly troublesome when attempting to relearn self-care activities. Characteristically, the memory loss is for recent events, while distant events often remain clear in his memory. This makes it difficult to provide a plan of care since he forgets from one session to the next how to perform an activity such as putting on a sweater. For this type of problem, repetition and constant performance under supervision may make it possible for him to develop a habit pattern. This can be a slow and tedious process.

Impairment of attention span and concentration ability may make it almost impossible to sustain the effort required to complete a task in spite of a clear mind. He is easily distracted from the performance of an activity and then forgets what he is doing. Such a patient is ofttimes labeled as lacking in motivation.

He may have perceptual difficulties which specifically affect his ability to perform self-care activities. Distortion of body image and/or sensory loss can present a multitude of difficulties in the area of self-care. At times a patient will have return of motor ability and will appear to have a clear mind, but he may be completely unable to perform a dressing activity because of these impairments. One obvious manifestation of this phenomenon is the neglect of the affected side often encountered in the left hemiparetic.

Incoordination, a disturbance of motor function in which smoothness and precision of motion are disturbed, may handicap him in self-care. Since this precludes fine dexterity he may need assistance with certain activities or be able to do them with delay and frustration. Activities which are often affected by this are buttoning and fastening in dressing activities and the conveyence of food from plate to mouth during eating activities.

Body balance may be affected. This is due to a disorder of the normal postural reflex mechanism, sensory disturbances, spasticity, loss of selective movement patterns, or muscle weakness from lack of activity. This will have varying effects on activities such as turning in bed, coming from a lying to a sitting position, maintaining sitting balance, transfer activities, sitting tolerance, and standing balance.

Homonymous hemianopsia, a visual field loss, will cause difficulties in nursing management, if not identified. For example, the patient may be said to be unresponsive because he does not recognize visitors, relate to other patients or the staff or reach for things on his bedside stand. These people frequently bump into other patients or push their wheelchair into the wall. When this is known his unit is arranged within his visual field and equipment is properly placed to enhance his independence.

Language problems that often occur may complicate or limit goals. Language is necessary for conscious thought and ability to understand. Its impairment implies interference in thinking as well as in communicating. The patient may understand what is being said but be unable to find the words to express himself. He may understand only a part of a sentence or he may not understand what he hears even when said in short and simple sentences.

Another factor which causes concern for all is lack of judgment. The patient does not recognize his physical limitation and does things unsupervised which jeopardize his safety. He may have the necessary motor function to perform self-care activities but because of poor judgment cannot be allowed to attempt those with risk factors.

Keeping in mind that any of the above phenomena can be present and in various degrees, the program in self-care activities is then planned.

The program is divided into the following: (1) sitting tolerance, (2) wheelchair mobility, (3) transfer, (4) bathing, grooming, dressing and (5) eating.

Sitting Tolerance

At the time of admission the nurse finds out the length of time the patient has spent out of bed each day. Ordinarily, it is about an hour or two a day. A sitting tolerance of more than this is necessary for performing activities on the nursing unit as well as participating in therapy sessions. It also becomes involved in such things as feeding and bathing oneself. Feeding oneself demands more physical energy in bed than when sitting in a chair.

Sitting tolerance is one of the first goals attained and this is accomplished by increasing the periods of time he is out of bed each day. This must usually be done against and in spite of marked protest. After the first week he usually has developed an eight-hour tolerance. Some ptaients, however, who have had long periods of bed rest require much more time to reach the eight-hour level. Weakness and disturbances in body balance are the two major factors which inhibit sitting balance and tolerance. The nurse must be prepared to accept her share of verbal abuse in accomplishing the above because most patients fatigue easily at first but will not gain unless the schedule is kept.

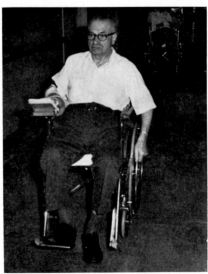

FIGURE 35. Patient manipulating wheelchair with nonaffected arm and leg. The foot is used for steering.

Wheelchair Mobility

Once he tolerates sitting for an adequate period of time, instruction in wheelchair mobility is begun. He learns to propel his wheelchair using his unaffected arm and leg. Several factors can influence his ability to functionally maneuver the wheelchair. The height of the chair seat will often keep a short person from touching the floor with his foot, a junior-sized chair may be necessary. Incoordination poses still another problem. Memory loss or receptive aphasia hinder his learning to manipulate the chair. He either forgets how or what he is doing or does not understand and/or carry through the instructions. Incoordination causes problems in momentum control and steering (see Fig. 35).

Transfer

When assisting in transfer activities it is important to remember that if the stroke is recent the patient is still adjusting to the changes in his body. He may not yet be able to adapt. Sitting is an example; he will fall to his affected side; also, he will tend to fall backward. To help offset this in transfer activities, he is instructed to put his chin down on his chest and bring his weight forward over his hips. He is always assisted from his affected side so that the ability to use his unaffected extremities is uninhibited (see Figs. 36-38).

There are several ways of placing the wheelchair in transfer activities. The most common method employed is as follows:

1. Place chair at slight angle to bed with unaffected side nearest to bed.
2. Lock brakes and lift up pedals.
3. Move unaffected foot close to wheelchair and grasp arm of the wheelchair.
4. Tuck in chin, push forward and up to standing position.
5. Get balance.
6. Move hand to bed.
7. Pivot one-quarter turn around.
8. Sit (see Figs. 39-43).

Transfer activities from chair to chair, chair to toilet, and so forth are performed in a similar manner. The following is the procedure used in tub transfer:

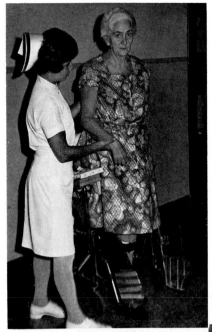

FIGURES 36-38. Basic transfer technique arising from a chair. Note assistance from affected side (see text).

FIGURE 36

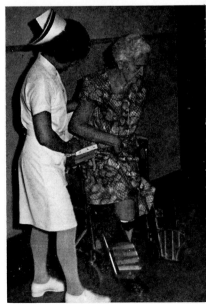

FIGURE 37

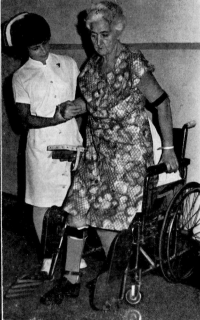

FIGURE 38

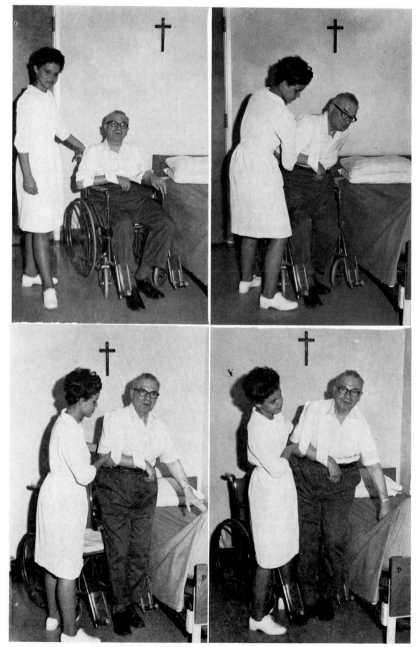

FIGURES 39-42

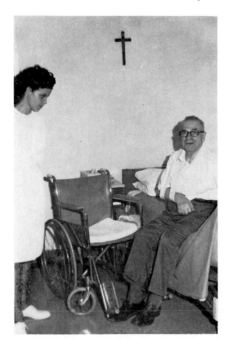

FIGURES 39-43. Chair to bed transfer (see text). When this and
reverse transfer have been mastered
a basic step in independence has
been achieved.

FIGURE 43

FIGURE 44. Bathtub equipped with
safety aids. Note right-angled bar
around back and front, slip-x strips
on the bottom, bathtub seat, and
grab bar on near side.

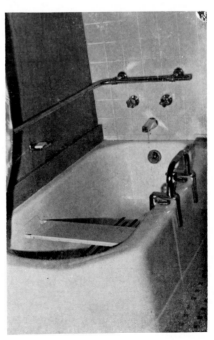

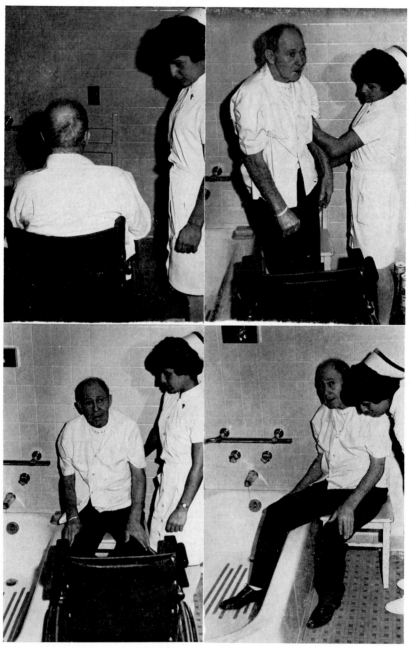

FIGURES 45-48

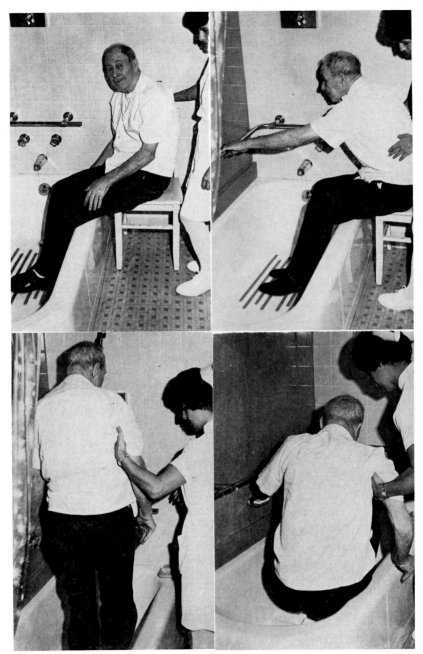

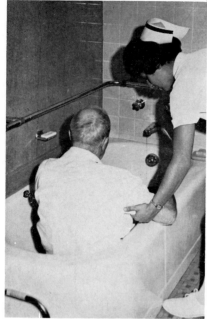

FIGURE 45-53. Tub transfer into tub (see text). Safety aids described in Figure 44 and assistance are necessary for it to be successful.

FIGURE 53

To prevent slipping, nonskid strips are placed in the tub. A wall grab bar on the far side of the tub and extending at a right angle around one end is essential (see Fig. 44).

1. For a right hemiparetic, place wheelchair parallel to tub with patient facing the end with the faucets. Place a straight chair without arms with its back against the wall parallel to the tub and facing away from the faucets toward the patient.

2. Patient stands from wheelchair, pivots, and sits in straight chair (see above).

3. Place affected leg into tub.

4. Lift unaffected leg into tub.

5. Grasp wall bar with unaffected hand.

6. Pull forward and up to standing position.

7. Turn and face faucet.

8. Assistant helps patient lower self into tub or onto bathtub seat (see Figs. 45-53).

The procedure is the same for a left hemiparetic except the unaffected leg goes in first and after standing, the patient slides his right hand along the wall bar and around the right angle while turning to sit.

The above description represents the safest way to perform tub transfer. In most cases assistance is necessary and advisable. In some home situations, such a transfer may be impossible and a simple transfer from chair outside tub to chair inside tub utilizing a rubber shower attachment for bathing may be the best solution.

To transfer the patient back into the chair from the tub the following steps are taken:

1. The assisting person places grab bar on near side of the tub and patient flexes knees so that feet are flat on bottom of tub.
2. Patient grasps side-wall bar and pulls himself forward and up with the help of the assistant.
3. Get balance.
4. Pivot to left, sliding nonaffected hand along side-wall bar, around the corner and along front-wall bar.
5. Transfer hand to grab bar on near side of tub.
6. Continue pivot to left and get balance.
7. Sit on chair with assistance.
8. Place unaffected leg outside of tub.
9. Lift affected leg outside of the tub (see Figs. 54-59).

If the patient is a left hemiparetic, he uses the grab bar on the near side of the tub to pull himself forward and up with assistance. He then reaches for the front-wall bar and pivots to the right and sits on the chair. The affected leg precedes the nonaffected leg out of the tub in this instance.

Bathing, Grooming, and Dressing

When the bathroom is used, the appropriate articles are made available. Soap, face cloths, towels, toothbrush, toothpaste, razor, and any other equipment which he needs are placed within his reach. If arrangements are such that these articles are in an accessible location, the patient can be independent. Otherwise, the nurse gathers the articles and puts them back in their proper place after use. Mirrors must be placed at levels accessible to wheelchair patients. If the bathroom is not large enough to accomodate a wheelchair, a regular chair, preferrably sturdy

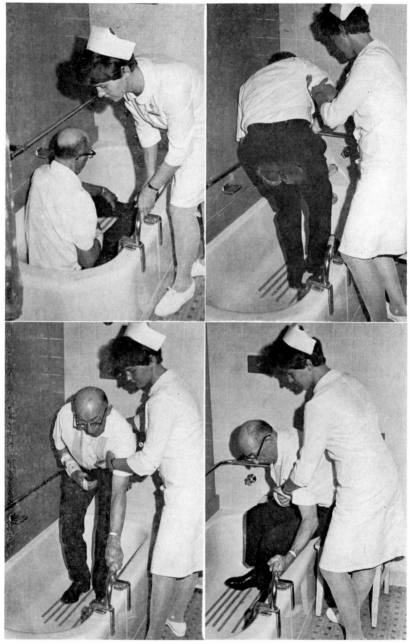

FIGURES 54-57

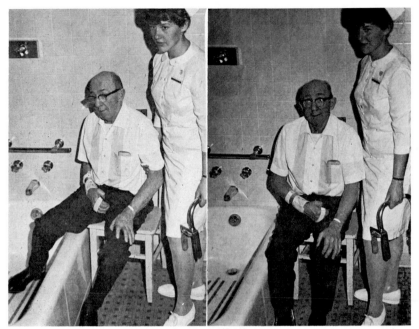

FIGURES 58-59
FIGURES 54-59.   Tub transfer out of tub (see text).

and with arms, can be placed at the sink for the patient to
sit on while caring for his personal hygiene.

Bathing is a simple task to normal people, but to the person
with a cerebral vascular accident it can seem insurmountable.
Therefore even though the nurse encourages independence, it
is still her responsibility that proper hygiene is maintained. In
many instances she will have to supplement his efforts. Usually
he is able to cleanse his face, neck, affected arm, and upper torso,
but many times he must be reminded to wash thoroughly. He
will need assistance with his unaffected arm if the affected arm
is nonfunctional.

Difficulty in body balance, weakness, interruption in body
image, memory loss, hemianopsia, impairment of sensation again
can cause him much difficulty. If there is distortion in body
image he will not care for that portion of his body of which he
is unaware. A homonymous hemianopsia will result in missing
the portions of his body which are not within his visual field. If

he has difficulty with his balance it will make bending to care for his legs and feet a hazard. He can lose his balance and topple forward out of his chair.

Tub baths are given at least once weekly and more often if deemed necessary. The use of a deodorant is important for both men and women. Many times it is easier to apply a roll-on type or a cream rather than the spray kinds which are sometimes difficult to manipulate.

Above all, the thing which can create more mental anguish is the lack of respect for the patient's privacy which is often neglected in the nurse's desire to get things done quickly.

The choice of clothing is important for the person who is learning to dress using one hand. There are certain styles, fabrics, and fasteners which make it easier to dress and to care for clothing than others. The following are some suggestions to use when selecting attire. During the initial learning period it is better to purchase inexpensive clothing. As the patient becomes more adept at dressing, better grades of clothing can be obtained.

Materials
    wrinkle resistant
    wash and wear variety
    seersucker
Slacks or trousers
    loose fitting (avoid tapered legs)
    high crotch
Dresses
    shift
    a-line
    dress with blouse top (removes strain from armholes)
    fullness in blouse such as pleats, gathers, or yoke-back (gives
       more width across back and prevents pull)
Blouse or shirts
    fullness such as pleats, gathers, or yoke-back
    cardigan type with large buttons
Skirts
    a-line
    gored
    circular cut
    pleated
    (avoid tight straight skirts—tend to ride up when sitting)
Slip
    half slip

regular with elastic inserts in straps
Underpants
    nylon type rather than cotton (slide easier)
    so-called snuggies should be avoided because are more difficult
        to put on
    elastic band should have give to it
Socks
    lightweight cotton without elastic tops
Shoes
    firm supporting oxford type
Laces
    zipper laces
    elastic laces
Sweaters
    cardigan with large buttons
    slip-on sweaters should be avoided

There are certain points which the nurse must be aware of when starting one-handed dressing activities:

1. The affected extremity is always dressed first. When undressing, clothing is first removed from the unaffected extremity.

2. Simple verbal instructions are given.

3. Instructions are repeated as often as necessary and always using the same words.

4. Verbal instructions and/or demonstrations may be necessary.

5. Clothing should be placed within easy reach.

6. Give him recognition each time he does something correctly. Never punish him by becoming angry with him.

7. The type of clothing chosen is important. There are styles, kind of material, etc., which can either help or hinder him in dressing.

8. There are many factors which can retard his ability to perform these activities.

9. The techniques are adapted to meet the needs of each person. Each person does not dress in exactly the same manner as another.

10. If a patient has difficulties following directions refer him to the head nurse for team evaluation.

Underpants, Pedal Pushers, and Trousers

Procedure for Dressing. *Method one*: Lying on a partly

raised gatch bed. Bend the affected leg and work the garment on up to the knee. The affected leg may be crossed over the bent good leg to prevent affected leg from slipping. Straighten affected leg and insert good leg. Work the garment up onto hips as far as possible. With good leg bent, press down with foot and shoulder to elevate hips from bed and pull garment up over hips. Or garment may be worked over hips by rolling from side to side, pulling garment up on the elevated side.

Method two: Sitting in a locked wheelchair with foot pedals in a down position. Move good leg over to midline of body. Lift affected leg with good hand and cross it over the good leg so legs are crossed. Slip garment up on to affected leg as far as the knee but *not* over it. Uncross legs and insert good leg into garment. Pull garment up legs as far as possible. Swing foot pedals into an up position. Stand and pull garment up over the hips. To prevent garment from dropping as the patient stands, the fingers of the affected hand may be slipped into the pocket, into the belt loop, or twisted into the elastic top. Sit down and fasten garment.

PROCEDURE FOR UNDRESSING. *Method one*: Lying down in partly raised gatch bed. Unfasten garment. Hips are hiked as in putting garment on in method one. Garment is worked down past hips, unaffected leg is removed, then affected leg.

Method two: Sitting in a locked wheelchair with foot pedals up. Unfasten garment and work it down the hips as far as possible. Stand and let garment drop past hips. Sit down, swing foot pedals down, remove garment from unaffected leg. Cross affected leg over good leg, remove garment.

Brassieres

PROCEDURE FOR DRESSING. With good hand, slide the bra behind the back at waist level. Fasten the hooks. Slip the fastened bra around the waist into correct position. Place the affected arm through the shoulder strap. Pull the strap up as far as possible on the shoulder. Slide the good hand through its shoulder strap and pull strap up into position. Adjust garment.

Comment: Elastic insert should be added to straps to ease the stress.

Procedure for Undressing. With good hand unfasten hooks and pull garment off.

Pullover Undershirts, Shirts, and Slips

Procedure for Dressing. *Method one*: Garment is positioned on lap, bottom toward chest and label facing down. With good hand, roll or gather up bottom edge of garment back all the way to the arm opening on affected side. Position arm opening as large as possible on lap and leave it there. Using good hand, place affected arm into opening and pull garment onto arm past elbow. Insert good arm. Adjust shirt on involved side up and onto shoulder. Gather garment back with good hand, lean forward, duck head and pass garment over head. Adjust the garment.

Comment: Slip straps may be lengthened with a two-inch piece of elastic to prevent them from breaking under stress.

Method two: Shake garment free of twists. Place on lap, front down and neck opening away from body. Gather up the back bottom of garment with good hand. Duck the head forward and pull garment over head. Reach up the opposite sleeve with good hand, grasp the affected hand and pull the affected arm through the sleeve. Slip the good arm through its sleeve and adjust garment.

Procedure for Undressing. If garment is long, stand and pull the garment up around hips with the good hand. Sit down. Starting at the top back, gather garment up in good hand, lean forward, duck head, and pull garment over head. Remove from good arm and then from affected arm.

Blouses, Shirts, Coats, and all Cardigan Garments

Procedure for Dressing. Shake the garment free of twists. Using good hand, place affected hand into its sleeve opening. Pull garment up over arm until shoulder is in place. Reach behind body with good hand and put into its sleeve, raising arm up to "shake" sleeve into position past the elbow. Line up garment front for buttoning.

Comment: If cuff on unaffected side is fastened with a button do one of the following:

1. Button before putting garment on and work good hand through the fastened cuff. If opening is too small, sew button on with elastic thread.

2. Button with a button hook attached to table with a suction cup.

3. Sew small pieces of Velcro to inside of cuff. Roll wrist on solid surface to fasten. NOTE: Velcro tends to collect lint which decreases its ability to adhere. Light brushing of both pieces will remove the lint. Close both pieces when washing.

PROCEDURE FOR UNDRESSING. *Method one*: Unbutton garment. Lean forward and make sure garment is free in back. With good arm, gather garment up in back of neck, duck head and pull material over the head. Remove garment from good arm and then from affected arm.

Method two: Unbutton garment. With good hand, throw shirt off good shoulder. Pull down cuff on unaffected side with good hand. Sleeve is worked off by intermittently shrugging shoulder and pulling down on cuff. Lean forward, bring garment across the back and remove from affected arm.

Comment: If cuff of sleeves are buttoned, the sleeve of the good arm may be unfastened in the following ways:

Grasp the side edge of the sleeve cuff between your teeth. Pull until button is in center of button hole. Lift arm to fold cuff back over itself and pull outward. Button should slide out.

Unfasten using a button hook attached to a table with a suction cup.

Unfasten Velcro by rubbing it against body.

Socks or Stockings

PROCEDURE FOR DRESSING. Sitting in locked wheelchair with foot pedals down. Bring good leg to midline of body. Lift affected leg across it. Top of stocking is opened by inserting the thumb and first two fingers near top and spreading them apart. Stocking is slipped over toes and half way down foot. The rest of the stocking is gathered onto the foot by gently pulling on first one side, then the other. Slide stocking around on foot until heel is in correct alignment. Pull gathered stocking up over heel. Work stocking up leg by gently pulling first on one side then the other.

PROCEDURE FOR UNDRESSING. Slide stocking down leg as far as possible. Cross affected leg over good leg. Slip the stocking down over heel and pull off.

Short-leg Brace

PROCEDURE FOR DRESSING. Sitting in a locked wheelchair with the foot pedals down. Fold T-strap down so it is caught behind the upright bar. Pull the opening as large as possible and fold the tongue back out of the way. Bring the good leg to midline of body and lift the affected leg across it. Hold the brace by the top of the inside upright bar. Swing brace back behind foot and forward so the heel is between the bars and toes inserted into the shoe opening as far as possible. If toes catch in edge of shoe, twist the brace so the shoe opening is at a slight angle before inserting toes. Hold the brace in position with pressure on the outside upright bar between the legs. Insert the shoehorn behind the heel as far down in shoe as possible. Hold top of inside upright bar and uncross affected leg. Place on foot pedal of wheelchair. Press down on knee with good hand until foot slips into shoe. If the patient complains that his toes are curled inside the shoe or if the foot does not slide readily into the shoe, lift the affected leg off the foot pedal by pulling up on the top of the inside upright bar. Kick the foot pedals into up position with good leg. Place both feet in good position on floor. Stand. Pressure of standing will ease the curled toes and slide the foot into the shoe. When sitting with foot pedals down, fasten top strap, then T-strap, then shoe.

PROCEDURE FOR UNDRESSING. Sitting in locked wheelchair with foot pedals down. Cross affected leg over good leg. Unfasten shoe and straps. Push down on inside upright bar until shoe is off foot.

Miscellaneous

SLINGS. While sling is lying on lap or table, buckle strap in back of arm support. Put sling over head, reach through sling with good hand, grasp affected arm and pull it through into sling. The elbow should be at the back of the sling and the wrist should be supported.

SHAVING. Use an electric razor. The skin or the cheeks can be made taut by blowing air into them with the mouth closed.

Cutting Fingernails. An ordinary nail clipper and fingernail file can be used by the good hand in caring for the nails on the affected hand. A leather and elastic holder for the nail file will secure the nail file in the affected hand. The nails of the good hand can then be filed and cleaned.

Eyeglasses. Place glasses on lap with curve of stem pointed up and the nosepiece down. Secure with hand of affected arm. Clean with good hand.

Shoe Fastening. Insert permanent plastic zippers (see Fig. 60).

Washing Uninvolved Hand and Arm. A suction cup brush is secured to side of washbowl where it can easily be soaped and rinsed (see Fig. 61). The good hand and forearm is rubbed over the brush. Any regular long-handled bath brush can be manipulated by the good hand to wash the good upper and underarm.

Drying the Uninvolved Hand and Arm. Spread two or more paper towels in the lap or catch the paper towels or a regular towel under the belt. Rub the hand over the towels until dry. Catch the regular towel over the towel rack. Rub the upper arm over the secured towel until dry.

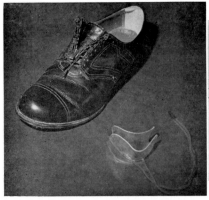
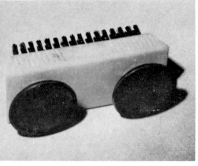

Figure 60.   Inexpensive zipper shoe lacing which can be laced into regular shoes. Note plastic shoehorn which is molded to each specific shoe.
Figure 61.   Suction brush which may be used to wash hand and forearm.

Eating

This is an activity in which the patient can gain independence with relative ease. Usually he needs assistance with cutting meat, buttering bread, and pouring liquids, but with time and instruction he probably will become independent in these activities also.

The usual eating implements are provided unless he appears to need some additional assistance. The three most popular

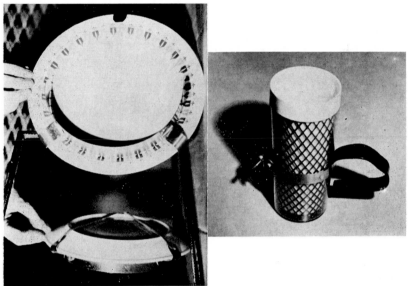

FIGURE 62. Plate guard which allows patient to push loose vegetables against it to load fork or spoon.
FIGURE 65. Removable handle for a glass.

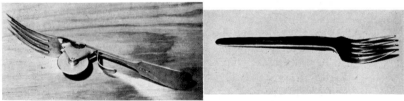

FIGURE 63. Fork with round cutting wheel which is utilized to cut meats with one hand.
FIGURE 64. Fork with cutting edge on one side. It is made for either left or right hand.

pieces of assistive equipment are the plate guard, fork-knife combination, and the removable handle for glasses (see Figs. 62-65).

He may have difficulty working the food onto his fork or spoon. The plate guard helps by providing a stable back against which to push the food. The combination of the knife and fork provides both the cutting and conveying implement in one.

He may have difficulty getting the food from the plate to his mouth. This can be due to either muscular weakness or incoordination but usually it is because of the former. The spoon handle can be bent to help offset this. Rather than use a cup, a handle can be added to his glass which permits him to handle the glass independently or with minimal supervision. One should remember that this type of equipment is only temporary and in many instances he will be able to use regular eating utensils.

The charge to the nurse may seem simple because it encompasses all of those daily routines which are done so routinely by well people. However, her task is fraught with problems, pitfalls, and personalities. The former routine process of putting on a shirt or blouse can now seem insurmountable to the individual who has lost the use of one upper extremity.

The nurse must be not only teacher and friend but she must also be generously endowed with patience, tolerance, humor, tenacity, knowledge, kindness, gentleness, understanding, and love.

REFERENCES

A Handbook of Rehabilitative Nursing Techniques in Hemiplegia. Minneapolis, Kenny Rehabilitation, 1964.

ANDERSON, HELEN: Stroke: Some nursing responsibilities. *Cardio-Vascular Nurs, 1*:1, 1965.

BOBATH, BERTA: Observations on adult hemiplegia and suggestions for treatment. Reprint from *Physiotherapy,* December 1959 to January 1960.

BORDEN, WALTER: Psychological aspects of stroke: Patient and family. *Ann Intern Med, 57:*

BRUNNSTROM, SIGNE: Walking preparation for adult patients with hemiplegia. *J Amer Phys Ther Assoc, 54*:17, 1964.

COVALT, NILA: Preventive techniques of rehabilitation for hemiplegic patients. *Gen Prac 17*:131, 1958.

CRAWFORD, MYRTLE, AND HEIEREN, ELEANOR: Rehabilitation in a teaching program. *Canad Nurse, 55*:201, 1959.

DAVIDSON, ROBERT: The psychologic aspects of strokes. *Geriatrics, 17*:151, 1963.

DILLER, LEONARD: New insights into the psychological problem. *J Rehab, 29*:41, 1963.

DRAKE, MELBA: Rehabilitation: An added dimension in nursing care. *Amer J Nurs, 60*:1105, 1960.

FISCHER, HERBERT, AND WEISS, HERMAN: Rehabilitation of the hemiplegic patient. Reprint from the *Illinois Medical Journal,* 1962.

FOWLES, BETH: *Syllabus of Rehabilitation Methods and Techniques.* Cleveland, Stratford Press, 1963.

HARTIGAN, HELEN: Nursing responsibilities in rehabilitation. *Nurs Outlook, 11*:649, 1954.

HAWKINS, KENNETH: Role of the nurse in rehabilitation. *Canad Nurse, 52*:1005, 1957.

HIRSCHBERG, GERALD, et al.: *Rehabilitation: A Manual for the Care of the Disabled and Elderly.* Philadelphia, Lippincott, 1964.

HURD, GEORGINA: Teaching the hemiplegic self care. *Amer J Nurs, 62*:64, 1962.

KNAPP, MILAND: Problems in rehabilitation of the hemiplegic patient. *JAMA, 159*:224, 1959.

KNAPP, MILAND, AND OWEN, RICHARD: Rehabilitation of the hemiplegic patient. *Geriatrics, 14*:306, 1959.

MacDONALD, JOANNE: An investigation of body schema in adults with cerebral vascular accidents. *Amer J Occup Ther, 14*:75, 1960.

MATTINGLY, CAPOLITA: Effective nursing for the stroke patient. *J Rehab, 29*:30, 1963.

MORRISSEY, ALICE: Rehabilitation in hemiplegia—Major nursing functions. *Amer J Nurs, 62*:58, 1962.

MORRISSEY, ALICE: *Rehabilitation Nursing.* New York, Putnam, 1951.

PESZCZYNSKI, MIECŻYSLAW: The rehabilitation potential of the late adult hemiplegic. *Amer J Nurs, 63*:111, 1963.

RUSK, HOWARD, et al.: *Rehabilitation Medicine.* St. Louis, Mosby, 1958.

SPAIN, RUTH: Rehabilitation nursing for the long-term patient. *Rehab Lit, 25*:1, 1964.

STANTON, MERIBAH: A review of Literature Concerning Four Aspects of Nursing Care of Stroke Patients. Unpublished Master's thesis, Department of Nursing, Boston College, 1966.

TREANOR, WALTER, et al.: Selective re-education and the use of assistive devices. *Phys Ther Rev, 34*:618, 1954.

TURNER, GWENDOLYN: The cerebrovascular accident patient. *Nurs Outlook, 8*:326, 1960.

ULLMAN, MONTAGUE: *Behavioral Changes in Patients Following Strokes,* W. A. Selle, Ed. Springfield, Thomas, 1962.

ULLMAN, MONTAGUE: Disorders of body image after stroke. *Amer J. Nurs,* *64*:89, 1960.

UP AND AROUND: A booklet to aid the stroke patient in activities of daily living. Washington, Superintendent of Documents, U. S. Gov. Print.

WEPMAN, JOSEPH: *Recovery from Aphasia.* New York, Ronald, 1957.

WHITEHOUSE, FREDERICK: The nurse and her role in rehabilitation. *Rehab* *Rec,* July-August, 1962, p. 9.

Chapter VIII

ROLE OF THE PHYSICAL THERAPIST

THE RESPONSIBILITY OF the physical therapist begins as soon as the physician refers the patient for active participation in a physical therapy program. Ideally the therapist has also received written aims and orders from the physician by which to guide the planned program (see Chap. VI).

As soon as the patient has been assigned to and met the therapist who will supervise his program, he undergoes more specific evaluation.

Precise evaluation of the stroke patient and definition of needs are the keys to planning a successful treatment program. Evaluations are done not only upon admission of the patient, but at specified intervals during treatment and at the time of discharge. If possible, the patient should return one to two months following discharge for a follow-up evaluation so that his present level of function can be assessed.

The physical therapy department routinely uses the following tests in evaluating the hemiplegic patient: the functional test, muscle test, range of motion test, gross sensory test, and a brief evaluation of the patient's ability to manipulate a wheelchair and ambulate.

Bennett defines the functional test as an evaluation of the patient's ability to overcome physical obstacles encountered in a normal environment. This test gives an objective measure of the patient's abilities and disabilities. It can be used by the physician, physical therapist, occupational therapist, and rehabilitation nurse to structure and carry out an ADL (activities of daily living) ward program. It makes it possible to record progress, and often supplies information which justifies continuing or discontinuing treatment. It can demonstrate the value of an assistive device. Further the information may be helpful to the social worker in

97

planning for the patient's return home and to the vocational counselor in planning for reeducation, retraining, or work placement.

There is no standard form for a functional test. However, to be a useful tool in rehabilitation, a functional test must meet certain requirements. Each test must have a clear grading system that demonstrates degrees of progress. Each activity must measure what the patient can do by himself, without assistance, but with safety, and within a reasonable amount of time. The

CHART 1

FUNCTIONAL TEST FOR HEMIPLEGICS

LEFT _____

NAME _____ AGE____ DATE OF ONSET_____ RIGHT_____

APHASIA____ HEMIANOPSIA____ OTHER DISABILITY_____

*Scale: ■ = adequate performance
▨ = partial performance, functionally inadequate
☑ = performance impossible

DATE			COMMENTS
		I. SUPINE	
		1. Move from place to place in bed.	
		2. Turn onto left side.	
		3. Turn onto right side.	
		4. Raise heel of involved extremity off bed.	
		5. Extend hip and knee against resistance.	
		6. Internally rotate involved extremity.	
		7. Place both feet over edge of bed.	
		8. Sit erect from supine position.	
		9. Remain sitting, back unsupported.	
		II. SITTING, ON BED, MAT OR CHAIR WITHOUT ARMS	
		A. Neck and trunk	
		1. Flex neck from complete extension.	
		2. Extend neck from complete flexion.	
		3. Turn head to side.	
		4. Bend head to side.	
		5. Arms at sides, bend trunk to left.	
		6. Arms at sides, bend trunk to right.	
		7. Arms folded, turn trunk to each side.	
		8. Arms folded, lean forward and return.	
		B. Upper Extremity	
		1. Raise arm overhead.	
		2. Hand to mouth.	
		3. Hand behind back	
		4. Reach forward, straightening elbow.	
		5. Pronate - Supinate	
		6. Grasp and hold (medium and large objects).	

functional test should include all necessary items for daily living, and be applicable to the bed, wheelchair, and ambulatory patient. It is preferable for the test form to accomodate serial testing on the same sheet so as to reduce the total number of test forms within the patient's chart.

Many such forms become useless to the physical therapist because they attempt to include too many activities and thus become too time-consuming. An ideal test, therefore, must include all the necessary items, but at the same time remain practical and workable.

Most functional tests are set up to include any motor disability. The Functional Test for Hemiplegics herein discussed applies only to the stroke patient (see Chart 1).

CHART 1 (Continued)

DATE				COMMENTS
		7. Pinch (oppose thumb to index finger).		
		8. Straighten fingers with wrist neutral.		
		III. SITTING IN WHEELCHAIR		
		1. Transfer from bed to wheelchair and back.		
		2. Manage brakes.		
		3. Manage leg rests and/or pedals.		
		4. Propel wheelchair (any method).		
		5. Transfer to toilet and back		
		IV. STANDING IN PARALLEL BARS		
		1. Stand from wheelchair		
		2. Lift involved leg with knee flexed		
		3. Lift involved leg, place heel down first		
		4. Lift involved leg to side		
		5. Lift good leg		

ACTIVITIES OF DAILY LIVING

		1. Dress self		
		2. Feed self		
		3. Ascend and descend stairs		
		4. Ascend and descend ramp		
		5. Ascend and descend curb		
		6. Walk on rough surface		
		7. In and out of bathtub		
		8. On and off toilet, (from standing)		
		9. On and off chair without arms, (from standing).		

AMBULATION DEFICITS

DATE	MARKED	MODERATE	MINIMAL	NONE	
					Loss of balance; direction
					Hip drop
					Genu recurvatum
					Toe drag
					Supination of foot
					Hip adduction
					Knee in flexion in stance phase
					Variance in stride
					Weak push-off

The test has space for the date and performance of the activity tested as well as any pertinent comments. Performance is graded as either adequate, partial (functionally inadequate), or impossible, and is accomplished by pencil shading. Pertinent data including the patient's name, age, involved side, date of onset, etc., is included. The test evaluates the patient in the supine, sitting, and standing positions and judges the patient's ability to move from place to place. It also tests neck and trunk balance, strength, and mobility, and evaluates the ability of the affected upper and lower extremities to function against gravity in motions necessary for daily living. The Functional Test for Hemiplegics examines the patient's ability to utilize his wheelchair independently. Another part of the test checks the specific activities of daily living; dressing and feeding, transfer to toilet and armless chair, use of tub, and ability to negotiate curbs, ramps, and stairs. The final section of the test explores ambulation deficits; loss of balance, hip drop, *genu recurvatum,* toe drag, supination of foot, hip adduction, knee flexion in stance phase, variance in stride, and weak push-off. Each one of these deficits is then graded as nonexistent, minimal, moderate, or marked.

Once the functional test has been completed, a muscle evaluation test is done. This gives valuable information concerning the strength of specific muscle groups. It is based on the assumption that if certain muscles or a muscle group are paralyzed or weakened, some specific motion will be lost or weakened. The muscle test is therefore an evaluation of the measure of a person's ability to actively contract a muscle or group of muscles against a known resistance. This resistance can be manual or mechanical. Manual resistance utilizes gravity and manual pressure and involves subjectivity in assigning a strength grade. Mechanical resistance is more objective and can detect grade changes more rapidly. However, it requires more time and money and is used mainly in research.

The muscle test determines the site and distribution of weakness or paralysis of muscles. This information is used in choosing a particular type of exercise and permits the physical therapist to determine if an orthopedic device is necessary. Serial testing evaluates the type of treatment used and aids the physician in prognosticating the expected muscle return.

There is no standard muscle evaluation form, although most forms are based on the Lovett System devised in 1915 by Dr. Robert Lovett. This system employs gravity and manual resistance. Each muscle or muscle group is assigned a grade ranging from zero to normal following palpation and inspection of that muscle or muscle group as it is called on to actively contract. Precise palpation is required as the muscle contracts and relaxes to discover possible substitutions by other muscles.

A muscle receiving the grade "zero" exhibits no palpable or visible contraction and is unable to move the desired body part. A "trace" muscle gives a palpable contraction with no visible motion. A "poor minus" muscle is capable of incomplete range of motion with gravity eliminated, whereas a "poor" muscle can move the body part through full range with gravity eliminated. Muscles grading "poor plus" exhibit motion through 50 per cent or less of the desired range against gravity while a "fair minus" grade denotes 50 to 90 per cent range of motion against gravity. A "fair" muscle moves the body part through full range of motion against gravity.

At the fair plus level, a muscle is regarded as functional, for it is capable of full range of motion against gravity plus sustaining a fair amount of resistance. Likewise, a good muscle can withstand a good amount of resistance. A "good plus" muscle would denote moderate weakness, while a normal minus grade indicates slight weakness. Finally, a "normal" muscle is capable of taking a normal amount of resistance.

It is evident that a therapist can be more objective in assigning muscle grades from zero to fair. Once she finds herself giving grades of fair, good, and normal (with or without plus and minus signs), muscle testing becomes much more subjective. The resistance sustained by a muscle is the amount given manually by the therapist and also reflects the "good" or "normal" for the patient as regards to size, sex, age, and occupation.

The muscle test illustrated here is less specific than some forms as it concentrates on grading major muscle groups rather than a specific muscle within that group (see Chart 2). For the hemiplegic patient, this appears practical since one is more interested in discovering if the patient can raise his affected hand to his mouth utilizing elbow flexors rather than knowing if he does this motion with his biceps or brachioradialis muscles. When weakness is discovered in a muscle group, the therapist attempts to strengthen what is left, then, if necessary, encourage substitution of the weakened motion by other muscle groups.

Range of motion in the joints of affected extremities is next evaluated by the range of motion test. This provides a quantita-

CHART 2

MANUAL MUSCLE EVALUATION
Cardinal Cushing Rehabilitation Unit—Physical Therapy

Name:
Diagnosis:

Age:
Date:
Therapist:

Left				Date		Right		
			N	Flexors	N			
			E	Lateral Flexors	E			
			C	Extensors	C			
			K	Rotators	K			
			T	Flexors	T			
			R	R.Ext.Obl.•Rotators L.Ext.Obl.	R			
			U	L.Int.Obl. R.Int.Obl.	U			
			N	Extensors—Thoracic	N			
			K	Extensors—Lumbar	K			
				Quadratus Lumborum				
			S	Abductor—Serratus Ant.	S			
			C	Adductors—Middle Trapezius	C			
			A	—Rhomboids	A			
			P	Elevators—Upper Trapezius	P			
			U	—Levator Ang. Scap.	U			
			L	Lower Trapezius	L			
			A	Latissimus Dorsi	A			
			S	Flexors	S			
			H	Extensors	H			
			O	Abductors (ABD & Elevation	O			
			U	Adductors	U			
			L	Horizontal Abductors	L			
			D	Horizontal Adductors	D			
			E	External Rotators	E			
			R	Internal Rotators	R			
			EL	Flexors	EL			
			BOW	Extensors	BOW			
			FORE	Supinators	FORE			
			ARM	Pronators	ARM			
			W	Flexors—Radial	W			
			R	—Ulnar	R			
			I	Extensors—Radial	I			
			S	—Ulnar	S			
			T		T			
			F	Flexors—MP	F			
			I	Flexor—Proximal IP	I			
			N	Flexor—Distal IP	N			
			G	Extensor—MP	G			
			E	Extensor—Proximal IP	E			
			R	Abductors	R			
			S	Adductors	S			
				Opponens—Digiti Quinti				
			T	Flexor—MP	T			
			H	Flexor—IP	H			
			U	Extensor—MP	U			
			M	Extensor—IP	M			
			B	Abductors	B			
				Adductors				
				Opponens Pollicis				

tive evaluation of gross movement with reliability established through using goniometry.

The range of motion or lack of it in affected joints influences the physician in planning the patient's program. A precise diagnosis of the cause of lost range such as contracture, spasticity, edema, or pain must be made in order to plan the proper treatment. The physical therapist measures and records the motion range in the patient's affected upper and lower extremity in order to keep a baseline against which to compare progress. The

CHART 2 (Continued)

Left				Date		Right		
			H	Flexors	H			
			I	Extensors	I			
			P	Abductors	P			
				Adductors				
				External Rotators				
				Internal Rotators				
				Gluteus Medius				
				Sartorius				
				Tensor Fascia Latae				
			K	Flexor-Outer Hamstring	K			
			N	Flexor-Inner Hamstring	N			
			E	Extensors	E			
			E		E			
			A	Dorsal Flexors	A			
			N	Plantar Flexors	N			
			K	Gastrocnemius	K			
			L	Soleus	L			
			E		E			
			F	Invertor-Ant. Tib.	F			
			O	Invertor-Post. Tib.	O			
			O	Evertor-Peroneus Long.	O			
			T	Evertor-Peroneus Brev.	T.			
			H		H			
			A		A			
			L	Flexor	L			
			L	Extensor	L			
			U		U			
			X		X			
			T	Flexors	T			
			O	Extensors	O			
			E	Abductors	E			
			S	Adductors	S			
				GIRTH MEASUREMENTS				
			Thigh:	Inches above Prox. Patellar Border				
			Calf:	Inches below Distal Patellar Border				

KEY: N Normal: Complete range of motion against gravity with full resistance.
G Good: Complete range of motion against gravity with some resistance.
F Fair: Complete range of motion against gravity.
P Poor: Complete range of motion with gravity eliminated.
T Trace: Evidence of slight contractility with no joint motion.
O Zero: No evidence of contractility.
S Spasm:) If spasm or contracture limit range of motion, place C or S
C Contracture) after the grade of a movement incomplete for this reason.

COMMENTS:

serial range of motion test provides a powerful motivation tool for the patient as he can see himself improve. The therapist also can evaluate the results of treatment. These tests serve as objective records for interpretation by other nonmedical personnel such as insurance companies.

There are two general classifications of recording instruments used to measure range of motion. The first is a protractor with one or two movable arms so that the arms can be placed parallel to the anatomical lever arms of the joints. After the joint completes the motion, the two arms of the goniometer are aligned, and the center of the protractor locates itself over the axis of joint motion. This is the instrument in common practice today. The second classification covers all instruments which are used to measure particular joints.

CHART 3
JOINT MOTION MEASUREMENTS
Holy Ghost Hospital
Cardinal Cushing Rehabilitation Center

Name _____ Age____Unit No.____Therapist's_____
Initials

						Left/Right	Date							
A	P	A	P	A	P		Active or Passive Motion		A	P	A	P	A	P
						HIP	Flexion 0-125	HIP						
							Extension 0-10							
							Adduction 0							
							Abduction 0-45							
							Int. Rotation 0-45							
							Ext. Rotation 0-45							
						KNEE	Extension 0	KNEE						
							Flexion 0-140							
						ANKLE	Plant. Flexion 0-45	ANKLE						
							Dorsi Flexion 0-20							
						FOOT	Inversion 0-40	FOOT						
							Eversion 0-20							
						SHOULDER	Extension 0-45	SHOULDER						
							Flexion 0-180							
							Adduction 0							
							Abduction 0-180							
							Int. Rotation 0-90							
							Ext. Rotation 0-90							
						ELBOW	Extension 0	ELBOW						
							Flexion 0-145							
						FOREARM	Supination 0-90	FOREARM						
							Pronation 0-90							
						WRIST	Extension 0-70	WRIST						
							Flexion 0-80							
							Ulna Dev. 0-45							
							Radial Dev. 0-20							

NOTE: The anatomical position is considered zero, and is the starting position with the exception of:
1. Shoulder rotation (shoulder abduction to 90°)
2. Supination and pronation (elbow flexed to 90°)

Measurement forms may vary among physical therapy departments, but the goniometer and techniques of measurement are similar. The anatomical standing position is usually used as the starting point with the exception of the radioulnar joint which has a resting position of 90 degrees of supination (see Chart 3).

To measure the active range of elbow flexion, the patient is first placed in the supine position with the arm to be measured parallel to the midline of the body and the palm of the hand facing anteriorly. The stationary arm of the goniometer is placed along the lateral midline of the humerus directed toward the acromion process while the moving arm is placed along the lateral midline of the radius toward the styloid process. In this situation, the axis of movement is in the vicinity of the lateral condyle of the humerus.

CHART 3 (CONTINUED)

A	P	A	P	A	P		Date		A	P	A	P	A	P
							Active or Passive Motion							
						THUMB	Flexion – CMC	THUMB						
							Extension – CMC							
							Flexion – MCP							
							Extension – MCP							
							Flexion – 1 PH							
							Extension – 1 PH							
						FINGERS	2 MCP Flexion 2 MCP	FINGERS						
							Extension							
							PIP Flexion PIP							
							Extension							
							DIP Flexion DIP							
							Extension							
							3 MCP Flexion 3 MCP							
							Extension							
							PIP Flexion PIP							
							Extension							
							DIP Flexion DIP							
							Extension							
							4 MCP Flexion 4 MCP							
							Extension							
							PIP Flexion PIP							
							Extension							
							DIP Flexion DIP							
							Extension							
							5 MCP Flexion 5 MCP							
							Extension							
							PIP Flexion PIP							
							Extension							
							DIP Flexion DIP							
							Extension							
						NECK Approx.	Flexion $0°–30°$	NECK Approx.						
							Hyperextension $0°–30°$							
							Lateral bend $0°–40°$							
							Rotation $0°–30°$							
						TRUNK Approx.	Flexion $0°–90°$	TRUNK Approx.						
							Hyperextension $0°–30°$							
							Lateral bend $0°–20°$							
							Rotation $0°–30°$							
							(dorsolumbar)							

COMMENT:

Pronation of the radio-ulnar joint is measured with the patient either sitting or backlying with the elbow flexed to 90 degrees and the arm held close to the side of the body. The forearm should be unsupported and in the midposition. The goniometer's stationary arm is placed on the dorsal surface of the wrist parallel to the long axis of the humerus; and the moving arm, at the end of the executed motion, is placed along the dorsum of the wrist on a level with the styloid processes.

A brief sensory exam is done prior to the application of any type of heat to the affected side of a stroke patient. Negligence in noting areas of decreased sensitivity may lead to burns or ulcerations. The skin can be tested with hot and cold coins and should be compared with the nonaffected side.

If the patient is initially confined to a wheelchair, his proficiency in manipulating the wheelchair is ascertained. If some

CHART 4

EVALUATION SHEET
Wheelchair Mobility

1. Complete independence

2. Partial independence
    a. Needs help over obstacles and doors; can't lock opposite side; independent transfer.
    b. Difficulty steering; supervision in transfer.
    c. Assistance in management of brakes and foot pedals; assistance in transfer.

3. Complete dependence

CHART 5

EVALUATION SHEET

Ambulation
1. Completely independent with or without brace

2. Partial independence
    1. Independent with or without walking aid.
    2. Supervision.
    3. Assistance.

3. Inability to walk

KEY: red = initial; black = discharge; green = follow-up.

degree of ambulation is present, this is assessed. These two brief, but highly informative tests are added to an ADL evaluation sheet compiled by the nursing staff, a speech form completed by the speech therapist (when appropriate), and a work ability test judged by the physician-in-charge. This entire evaluation is done at the time of admission, at discharge, and at follow-up (see Charts 4-8).

The wheelchair evaluation grades the patient as being wheelchair independent (1), partially independent (2), or completely dependent (3). The grading within the subcategory (2) allows for three grades within that division (see Chart 4).

The form for evaluation of ambulation is also divided into three categories and contains three separate subcategories within the partial independence group (see Chart 5). The appropriate

CHART 6

EVALUATION SHEET

ADL Activities

I.   Complete independence

    A.   Dressing and grooming
- 1. All but shoe, sock, brace, and bra.
- 2. Above, plus underpants and slacks.
- 3. Assistance required for more than above; procurement and laying out.

    B.   Bathing
- 1. Can't wash nonaffected arm, back, and axilla of affected arm.
- 2. Above plus leg and foot.
- 3. Above plus affected arm.

II. Partial independence

    C.   Tub bathing
- 1. Safety aids required; tub filled.
- 2. Supervision.
- 3. Assistance.

    D.   Toilet
- 1. Can transfer with aids.
- 2. Supervision.
- 3. Assistance.

    E.   Feeding
- 1. Food presented to him; feeds self.
- 2. Feeds self except cutting meat and buttering bread.
- 3. Above plus more direct assistance; aids.

III. Completely dependent

CHART 7

EVALUATION SHEET

Speech

I. Expressive aphasia

    A. No defect

    B. Partial defects

        1. Speaks in sentences.

        2. Phrases; 50-word vocabulary; telegraphic speech.

        3. Responds with "yes" and "no" appropriately.

    C. Complete inability to express the spoken word

II. Understanding (mixed aphasia)

    A. No defect—responds correctly to all commands

    B. Partial defects

        1. Follow simple commands, if repeated.

        2. Can imitate motions or gestures.

        3. Inconsistent response.

    C. Complete inability to follow through on commands

III. Perseveration

    A. No defect

    B. Partial defects

        1. May perseverate on a word or idea.

        2. Some meaningful phrases and sentences.

        3. Jargon interspersed with some correct syllables.

    C. No intelligible speech—complete jargon

CHART 8

EVALUATION SHEET

Work Ability

A. No restrictions

	Previous job holders	Housewives
B. Partial restrictions	1. Change of job.	1. Duties with family assistance.
	2. Retraining.	2. Part-time homemaker.
	3. Sheltered workshop.	3. Full-time homemaker.

C. Full restrictions

    1. Physical.

    2. Mental (includes motivation, attention span, etc.).

    3. Both.

    4. Previous retirement.

Work ability—Assessment of physical, mental and emotional ability to hold down a full-time job determined by patient's previous occupation.

numbers are encircled in red for the initial evaluation, black for discharge, and green for follow-up. The form is dated and signed by the physical therapist in charge of the patient. It is important to note that the stroke patient is considered to be completely independent in ambulation even though he may require a short-leg brace.

When the thorough basic evaluation has been completed and recorded the treatment plan is devised.

As stated previously, all physical therapy procedures are carried out under the written orders of the physician. These orders are not only for specific treatment modalities, but also are accompanied by the aims to be accomplished during the course of treatment. While the physician establishes the initial aims, any of these may change, be eliminated, or new ones developed as the treatment progresses. It is usually the physical therapist who notes these changes when progress notes are written and calls them to the attention of the physician.

Physical therapy procedures as applied to the stroke patient are numerous, but this chapter will deal exclusively with the techniques more commonly used. Five major areas will be discussed as they apply separately to the affected upper and lower extremities.

THE AFFECTED UPPER EXTREMITY

Relief of Pain

The patient who experiences pain in the involved upper extremity often finds it difficult to cooperate in physical therapeutic measures designed to improve the status of this extremity. The pain is usually in the shoulder and due to attempts to increase limited motion. The latter is due to either contracture, shoulder separation, spasticity, or combinations of all. Pain relief must be accomplished if the extremity is to be effectively mobilized. Inability to control pain often makes it necessary to leave that area alone and concentrate on other parts of the program. Otherwise the ability or desire to cooperate may be so scuttled that the entire program is in jeopardy.

Hot wet packs are the treatment of choice for they appear to be more effective in decreasing pain, in reducing muscle spasm, and in preparing the area for further treatment. The amount of heat is controlled by layers of towelling which surround the pack. An elbow, forearm, or wrist can also be treated with hot packs, but if the hand is to be heated, the paraffin bath is preferred. Paraffin is another form of hydrotherapy employing conductive heating and may be applied to the hand by repeated immersion into a bath until a glove is formed. The hand is then wrapped in a towel. The bath combines mineral oil with block paraffin to lower the melting point and make hand dipping possible. The oil and paraffin are mixed in the following proportions: one part mineral oil to four parts paraffin. The temperature should be between 125° to 130° and can be measured by thermometer or estimated when upon cooling the surface begins to congeal. Paraffin, like the hot wet pack, tends to relieve pain and muscle spasm, soften the skin, and prepare it for treatment to follow. In applying any form of heat, precautions are followed to prevent burns, and heat is contraindicated in patients with areas of scar tissue, skin grafts, skin infections, or open wounds unless closely supervised by the physician.

Range of Motion

The responsibility of the therapist in joint range of motion

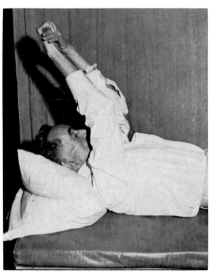

FIGURE 66. Patient performing range of motion of upper extremity.

is divided between maintaining normal range or restoring it when limited. During the first few days following a CVA, the affected upper extremity must be put through full range of motion at least six times daily. If time does not permit sufficient exercise, the patient whenever possible should be taught to use his unaffected arm to take the paralyzed upper extremity through gentle range of motion (see Fig. 66). At this stage many physical therapists will not have made contact with the patient, and it is essential that the nurse assume this duty. Early, while paralysis is complete, or if it persists, manual range of motion is also done passively by the therapist to prevent contractures from developing. It is preferable for passive range of motion to be done manually at this time, for it offers the therapist an opportunity to evaluate the areas of pain, spasticity, or site of possible contractures, and to develop a warm working relationship with the patient.

If the upper extremity does not regain muscle power, passive range of motion must be continued, even after the patient is

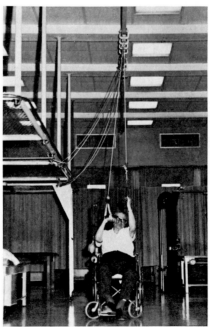

FIGURE 67.   Patient using overhead pulley to stretch shoulder contracture.

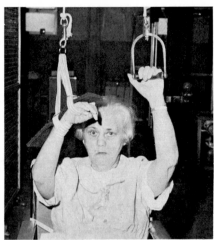

FIGURE 68.   Close up of sling arrangement for affected hand when using overhead pulley.

discharged from the hospital. While on the program, manual exercise continues, but a useful mechanical aid is introduced. The overhead suspension pulley provides another means for the patient to maintain his own range, utilizing the unaffected shoulder (see Figs. 67 and 68). Many patients enjoy the pulley apparatus, for this is one type of exercise where they are on their own, contributing to an important part of their program. They can also control the pain so induced. Since this exercise can be done without supervision, it is essential for the therapist to know that he can rely on the patient to do it properly. Combined with the self-exercises taught the patient for maintenance, the pulley is useful later for home exercises since it is cheaply and easily installed. If the patient is discharged home or to the home of a family member, an interested responsible member is often taught these same passive exercises so that he is prepared to supervise the patient or actually participate in giving them.

Unfortunately the majority of stroke patients referred for rehabilitation have well-established or early flexion contractures of the shoulder, and less commonly, contractures of wrists and fingers. When muscle contractures exist, selected stretching is indicated. Today, more emphasis is placed on selective stretching to obtain the amount of range of motion required for function.

This situation is best illustrated by a patient with a painful flaccid shoulder whose main requirement functionally is a shoulder that will flex and abduct sufficiently to allow him to dress and bathe. In the past, extensive stretching occurred without realizing that a mild contracture of a flaccid shoulder might be preferable to full range of motion. Nonfunctional hands that tend to curl or contain a moderate degree of spasticity are also fitted to simple static hand splints. If contractures of the wrist or fingers exist in this type of hand, they are stretched by the physical therapist so that proper alignment is possible in the splint. Selected stretching is also indicated because of the amount of pain the patient experiences. Even though the area is heated prior to stretching, it remains a painful part of the treatment program. Although once these contractures are stretched, patients are more comfortable, unlimited stretching, once function is obtained, is unjustified.

Three types of stretching exist: passive, active, and active-assistive. Most therapists utilize all three techniques to gain optimum results. In patients who are unable to cooperate, passive stretching is used exclusively. Active stretching is obtained by utilizing the overhead suspension pulley with well-motivated patients. Where active stretching is possible, the patient may be more inclined to push himself a bit farther in a set-up where he controls the amount of pain experienced rather than waiting and anticipating pain from the passive stretching of the therapist. Again, it must be emphasized that with active stretching, it is of the utmost importance that the patient be highly motivated and understand clearly what he is expected to accomplish.

An extremely useful and versatile apparatus for active and active-assistive stretching is sling suspension. This unit offers suspension of the desired part and provides for movement of the part free from gravity and friction. The suspension apparatus consists of an overhead and side frame which provide a multiplicity of fixation points plus ropes, various sizes of slings to support body parts, and springs which serve to assist or resist movement. One such apparatus, the Guthrie-Smith sling suspension unit, can be purchased from various hospital supply corporations. However, the general principles of suspension can be easily and inexpensively constructed by using a lightweight bedspring of the wire link type, supported on a Balkan frame, which is then secured to a hospital bed. It is adaptable to either hospital or home use. The author and staff have also developed a new portable sling suspension apparatus on locking wheels, made of aluminum and steel mesh screening. This is easily moved to wherever it is needed.

Regardless of the form used, sling suspension offers many advantages in its application. When the body part is suspended in slings, the force of gravity is counteracted. This is especially helpful with a painful contracted joint, for the patient feels secure in slings and begins to relax the tight spastic muscles about the joint. The patient need not worry that the physical therapist may accidentally drop the part or that he must support the part himself. Once relaxation begins, the patient can be instructed in mobilization exercises. The therapist's hands are free to direct or assist the desired movement. As the exercise begins, the patient appreciates that he alone is performing the movement since the therapist is not required to hold the part. Often, when manual support is given, the patient is unable to ascertain just how much he is capable of doing and how great is the contribution by the therapist. As the patient continues to work and the therapist is assured that the exercise is being carried out properly, he may leave the patient for periods of time to work on his own. This not only leaves the therapist more time for other patients, but has the effect of gradually building up the patient's confidence, since he is on his own to exercise, relax as he tires, then to begin again. Sling suspension gives one the opportunity to carry out not only the physical therapy procedures of increasing and maintaining range of motion, but also increasing and maintaining strength, and building endurance.

A number of sling suspension setups are useful in accomplishing the aims proposed for the stroke patient. For active shoulder stretching, a number of setups are possible, but the one most frequently employed places the patient sidelying with his affected upper extremity on top (see Fig. 69). The weakened arm is supported in two slings and suspended. This eliminates the need for the patient to be able to support his own arm against gravity and leaves the therapist's arms free for demonstration or assistance. The patient is encouraged to swing the arm as far as possible into flexion and extension.

A similar setup is utilized for mobilizing elbow flexion and extension and shoulder horizontal abduction and adduction. The patient sits in his wheelchair or on a straight chair while the upper extremity is supported at the shoulder and hand by slings. Once suspended in a relaxed position, the desired movements of the upper extremity are started (see Fig. 70). Sling suspension can also be utilized in the reeducation of muscles in the shoulder girdle.

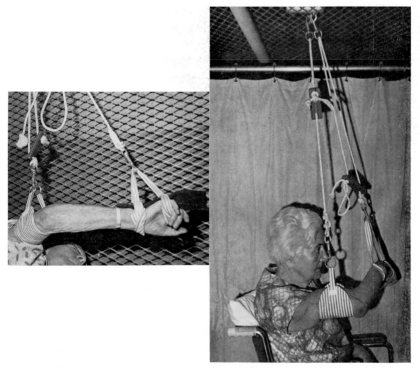

FIGURE 69. Patient in sling suspension, side lying position, performing active shoulder flexion and extension to increase range of motion.
FIGURE 70. Patient in sling suspension, sitting in wheelchair performing active horizontal abduction and adduction of shoulder.

Increase Strength and Endurance

As muscle power begins to return, various types of exercise are utilized to foster this return and strengthen the muscle groups. With active-assistive exercises, the patient executes the movement as best he can, and the therapist assists him in completing it. In this type of exercise, mechanical means may suffice as the assistance. Again, sling suspension may act in an assisting manner with proper placement of springs to complete a motion. Powder boards may be utilized so that the extremity is supported and friction diminished. Exercises are usually done in simple movement patterns, i.e. straight shoulder flexion, followed by straight shoulder extension. As the upper extremity improves in strength, the patient is next supervised in active exercise which involves eliminating assistance, but does not yet include resistance.

These active exercises are designed to maintain range of motion and foster strength of the affected upper extremity, utilizing the nonaffected side to assist the desired movements. Although the entire number of exercises should not be of such a number as to overwhelm the patient, each exercise should be detailed to permit as many essential movements as the patient can handle. For example, one exercise may include the motions of shoulder external rotation, elbow extension followed by shoulder flexion, shoulder horizontal adduction and abduction, and finally, elbow flexion and shoulder internal rotation. All these motions can be obtained if proper instruction and demonstration has been given to the patient.

When the extremity has improved to the point that it is capable of exercising against resistance, resistive exercises will be initiated by the therapist. If the arm is still quite weak (F+), it is preferable to give the resistance manually since certain areas of range can withstand less resistance than others. Mechanical resistance is utilized as soon as possible. Again sling suspension is utilized employing springs of various weights for resistance and progressive resistance exercise (PRE) (see Fig. 71).

Progressive resistance exercises are designed to obtain a rapid gain in muscle strength, bulk, and endurance. It should be stated, however, that PRE can also be used for muscles grading poor to fair in strength. This can be accomplished by counter-

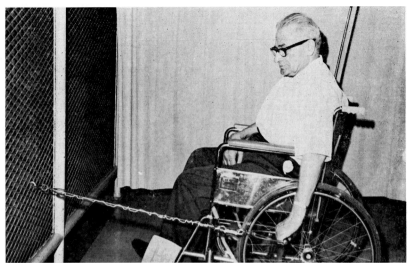

FIGURE 71. Patient performing shoulder extension in sitting position against spring resistance.

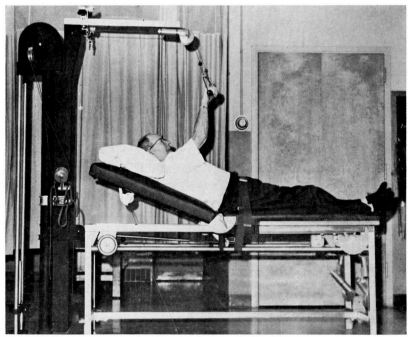

FIGURE 72. Patient performing load-assisted shoulder extension on Delorme table.

balancing the weight of the extremity with a cable and pulley arrangement to give a load-assisting rather than a load resisting exercise. A simple example can be illustrated with the Delorme table utilizing assisted shoulder extension (see Fig. 72). Once the strength of the extremity has surpassed the limitation of spring weights, regular weights are used.

In most physical therapy departments, the resistance or weight is lifted against gravity. The amount is initially determined by the maximum load the patient can lift ten times. Once the maximum is established, a total of thirty lifts is completed. The patient begins by lifting half the maximum load ten times, three-quarters the load ten times, then the total load ten times, resting three to four minutes between each load. Each load is lifted slowly, and the patient is encouraged to obtain full range of motion. Every few days an attempt is made to increase the load. Wall pulleys and barbells are used for shoulder, elbow, wrist, and finger strengthening.

If the therapist is primarily interested in increasing muscle endurance rather than strength, PRE is also important. Here, the load is not maximum and the number of repetitions or lifts is high.

Muscle reeducation is another type of exercise which cannot be isolated from the other forms. There are two types of reeducation procedures which employ quite different methods but attempt to accomplish the same end, i.e. to regain the ability to voluntarily contract a muscle or group of muscles.

The conventional type of muscle reeducation attempts to increase strength, endurance, and coordination of muscle groups by developing an awareness on the part of the patient for the desired motion. This is done through straight movements of each motion, i.e. straight shoulder flexion, then straight shoulder abduction. In this type, passive, active-assistive, resistive, and sometimes free active exercises are used to encourage the desired motion.

The second type of muscle reeducation is proprioceptive neuromuscular facilitation (PNF). PNF techniques attempt to make patient responses more spontaneous to handling. In other words, these techniques attempt to "hasten the response of the neuromuscular mechanism through stimulation of proprioceptors." Within this form of reeducation different schools exist, but basically they share certain main features. Maximal resistance is given to normal movement synergies whenever possible. Synergies are defined as basic movement patterns. These normal movement synergies are in diagonal or spiral patterns. Movements are made of the entire extremity, not just those which occur about a single joint. Stronger muscles are utilized to facilitate weaker ones. Resistance is given isotonically, isometrically, combined, and in certain patterns. For example, the therapist might choose to use repeated contractions. With this method of giving resistance, the patient moves the extremity through the strongest part of the range, holds the resistance isometrically, then completes the range. Concise instructions are given the patient, "pull—hold—pull." If the therapist were interested in fostering shoulder flexion, a mass movement would be attempted, bringing in thumb extension and adduction, finger extension and abduction, wrist supination and extension, forearm supination, shoulder abduction and external rotation, and scapular adduction and elevation. With these various patterns, therapists utilize body positioning, stretch reflexes, traction, and joint approximation in attempting to elicit these mass patterns of movements.

All stroke patients are not candidates for PNF, for many are unable to learn these patterns. With the existence of different schools of technique, most physical therapists borrow and combine various methods that they feel from their experience are of benefit. Both types of muscle reeducation are employed where appropriate, with specific patients.

Improved Coordination

Coordination has been defined as the ability to use the right muscles at the right time with the proper intensity to most efficiently achieve a desired movement. Physical therapists rarely receive primary orders from the physician to improve coordination or dexterity of the upper extremity. This responsibility is given to the occupational therapists who concentrate on the plegic or paretic hand. However the physical therapist participates in treating the shoulder. Coordination exercises are usually given with the patient in the supine position. One simple straight pattern is done at a time by the therapist, such as shoulder flexion with elbow extension. The patient is instructed to return the arm to the starting position. As the pattern is completed correctly, the therapist may ask for the same movement bilaterally, then progress to the point where each arm is simultaneously performing a different movement.

Reduce Spasticity

Spasticity is treated sometimes by the application of cold. Since research in this field is limited and no one claims to have discovered the most effective means of applying cold, each therapist chooses the method that he feels is most beneficial. Some prefer to use towels soaked in ice water, others apply the cubed or crushed ice wrapped in towelling directly to the part, while others prefer the prepared cold pack that is available commercially.

Even though cold is applied to a certain area or joint, it must be remembered that when more than a minimal amount is applied, the effects do not remain localized. The effect of cold is due to the use of one reflex (cold) to inhibit another (spasticity) since spasticity is based on hyperactive stretch reflexes. Through various studies, it has been demonstrated that the maximum reduction of spasticity occurs during the first minute of application even though the treatments may last ten to fifteen minutes.

Some patients have experienced maximum lasting relief while others have had none. It can be noted, however, that passive ROM (range of motion) or stretching of spastic muscles following a cold treatment is accomplished with greater ease. Occasionally, cold is applied to inhibit spastic flexors (most commonly of the elbow) while electrical stimulation is given to facilitate the extensors. This often releases more of an extensor response than could be obtained with the cold alone.

The system of treatment proposed by the Bobaths is also sometimes used by therapists trained in its performance. Primitive and exaggerated reflex activity is inhibited by holding various joints in the position opposite to that which they tend to assume.

For instance when one holds the spastic hand and wrist in extension when a patient is walking, the arm relaxes and the gait improves.

At times stroking select areas with a small brush will bring about relaxation of inhibitory muscle groups.

THE AFFECTED LOWER EXTREMITY

Relief of Pain

Contractures are seen less frequently in the lower extremity. The most troublesome is a knee flexion contracture, often caused by the injudicious use of a pillow. Also sitting too long with the knee flexed will encourage this deformity. Pain can be present in stiff contracted ankles and hips but it appears to resolve more easily. Hot packs are used with the same cautions as expressed above. In rare instances cold has been found to be more effective than heat.

Range of Motion

Much stated above in reference to the upper extremity is also applicable to the lower extremity. Passive range of motion exercises must be instituted on the paralyzed or very weak lower extremity as soon as possible to maintain full range. As weeks elapse without return of active muscle power, it will still be necessary to continue these exercises to prevent contractures, otherwise proper fitting of an orthetic device and the attainment of as near normal a gait as possible may be negated. The best way to prevent contractures from developing in the lower extremity is to foster early ambulation, proper positioning when the patient is in bed, as well as passive exercise to these areas.

If contractures develop, knee flexion occurs most often followed by hip flexion and external rotation and ankle plantar flexion. Hip and knee flexion contractures are usually produced by faulty positioning in the early stages such as placing a pillow under the knee for comfort or by failing to use a footboard. In some instances when a footboard is used, the soles of the feet only rest against the board, and the knees are flexed. The lack of a footboard or its improper placement, combined with

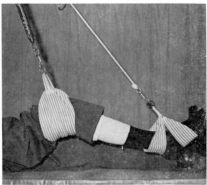

FIGURE 73. Patient in back lying position utilizing sling suspension and spring resistance to stretch knee flexion contracture.

infrequent ambulation also enhances the possibility of an ankle plantar flexion contracture.

Again, selective stretching is indicated. While it is usually important to decrease a heel cord contracture to improve gait and fit of a short-leg brace, in other specific situations mild contractures can be advantageous. For example, with a spastic hemiplegic, unable to relax the calf muscles during ambulation, a mild hip external rotation contracture helps to reduce the amount of resistance exerted by the calf in the stance phase of ambulation as the patient begins to lean forward.

Sling suspension is particularly useful for prolonged stretching. Slings are utilized to suspend the lower extremity while the patient actively pushes the contracted knee into extension against the resistance of springs (see Fig. 73).

Increase Strength and Endurance

Strengthening of the affected lower extremity proceeds in a similar fashion to the upper extremity. Active-assistive, active, then resistive exercises are utilized as the particular muscle or muscle group begins to return and increase in strength. Where applicable, the two types of muscle reeducation methods are employed from the very beginning of treatment.

For the very weak muscle, sling suspension with or without spring resistance is first utilized. The patient is placed in the supine position with slings under thigh and ankle to do hip abduction and adduction. The side lying position with the affected extremity uppermost is used for hip flexion and extension. Graduated spring resistance is introduced as muscle power increases.

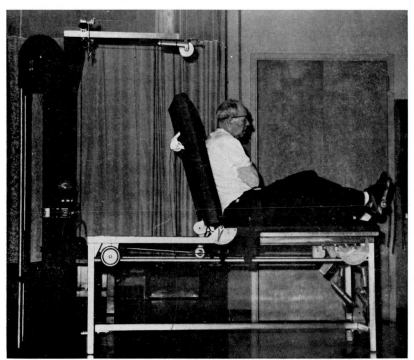

FIGURE 74. Resisted hip and knee extension on Delorme table.

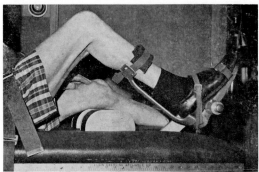

FIGURE 75. Close-up view of resisted hip and knee extension on Delorme table.

The patient progresses to the Delorme table where hip and knee extensors continue to be strengthened utilizing the advantage of counterbalancing the extremity with a cable and pulley arrangement (see Figs. 74 and 75).

When appropriate, the angle of flexion, the length of excursion, and the resistance are controlled and varied by the physical therapist. If endurance is preferred over strength, the resistance is reduced from maximum and more repetitions are required from the patient. This type of resistive exercise is also popular with the patient since he is aware of the amount of weight pushed each day and easily is aware of progress and proud of it.

The quadriceps boot is next employed and is highly useful and popular with patients (see Fig. 76). It helps to further increase strength and/or endurance of the knee extensor group so essential for ambulation. Here, any amount of resistance

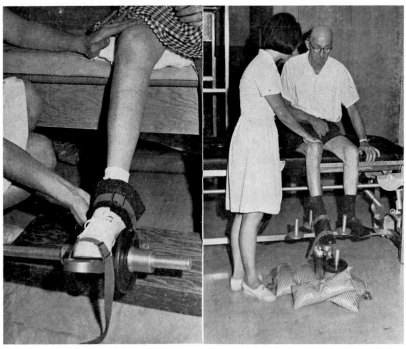

FIGURE 76.   Use of quad boot and weights for strengthening lower extremity.

FIGURE 77.   Delorme ankle exerciser.

can be employed and is carried out using the 10-RM system previously discussed.

The Delorme ankle exercisor is beneficial in strengthening ankle dorsiflexors, invertors, and evertors (see Fig. 77). This piece of equipment at times requires stabilization of its base with sandbags to prevent movement and substitution of knee action for ankle action.

Improve Coordination

In the lower extremity poor coordination is translated into a balance problem. This may range from a mild defect to marked instability which prevents functional ambulation or even transfer. A mild problem is treated by means of weight shifting in the standing position, utilizing the parallel bars. To begin, the affected foot is placed before the nonaffected foot and the weight shifts from front to back. Later, the normal foot is placed in

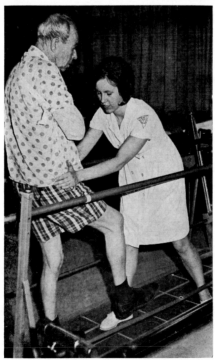

FIGURE 78. Performance of resisted gait by patient and therapist.

front and attempts are made to widen the stance. Weight shifting is also done from side to side with attempts to widen the base.

Resisted gait in and out of the parallel bars is also utilized for improving balance (see Fig. 78). The therapist manually resists the motion of walking. The resistance is usually given at the level of the pelvis and varies depending on the extent of the problem. This is one effective way of providing maximum stimulation to the balance receptors, and is suited to the patient with a mild or moderate balance defect. Resistance is given in forward, backward, and sideways directions.

Another effective method of giving maximum stimulation is rhythmical stabilization. This type of balance exercise can be given to the mildly involved patient in the standing position or the markedly involved individual on a mat or in the wheelchair. Rhythmical stabilization employs isometric contractions of all muscle groups about a joint and may be performed at any point in the range. Since it is a form of proprioceptive neuromuscular facilitation, it is dependent on maximum resistance to all movement patterns to elicit the desired isometric contractions. Trunk flexion and extension, as well as lateral movements of the trunk are the main areas of focus with the hemiplegic. These lateral movements become extremely important, especially with the severely spastic hemiplegic who exhibits a strong tendency to fall to the affected side.

When marked balance problems exist, they must receive at least equal or even more attention than weakness in order to achieve maximum rehabilitation.

Reduce Spasticity

Fortunately, in the experience of the authors, spasticity has not been as severe a problem in the lower extremity as that seen in the upper. It may contribute to a hazardous ungainly gait but it is not usually the primary cause for nonambulation.

The treatment methods discussed above which include the use of cold, electrical stimulation to the antagonists, and techniques of inhibition of abnormal reflexes are also used for the lower extremity. Unfortunately results obtained are not universally good or reproducible.

A more direct approach to the relief of spasticity has been

used by some. Peripheral nerve blocks with phenol have been successfully reported. Also surgical procedures have been devised which produce deafferentation of objectional regions responsible for massive proprioceptive inputs.

THE UNAFFECTED SIDE

No rehabilitation program is complete without an evaluation of the unaffected upper and lower extremity to determine any necessary areas for treatment. These areas are examined for pain, contractures, incoordination, spasticity, or weakness that may interfere with the patient's goal of independence. The most common deficit found is weakness due to prolonged bed rest. Good muscles have atrophied from disuse. In this situation, the physical therapist would develop an exercise program designed to strengthen all extremities. Occasionally the patient has had a previous stroke on the opposite side and more complications are evident.

WHEELCHAIR MANAGEMENT

For early independence, a nonambulatory patient must be capable of managing a wheelchair. Wheelchair management

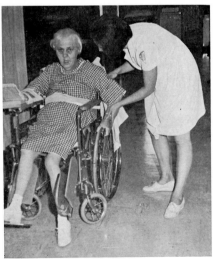

FIGURE 79. Instruction in propelling wheelchair using nonaffected arm and leg.

involves not only wheeling a straight line and around corners, but ability to get over thresholds, lock and unlock brakes on both sides, raise and lower foot pedals, and transfer. The stroke patient has a unique problem in accomplishing these requisites; he must learn to propel the chair (in most cases) with only his unaffected arm and leg (see Fig. 79). In addition he may be called upon to lock the brakes on his affected side with the normal upper extremity. He must be able with the normal arm to lift his affected leg on and off the foot pedal. His balance must be adequate for transfer and for bending to raise and lower the foot pedals.

The patient is introduced to wheelchair activities by the rehabilitation nurse as soon as mobilized from bed unless he has immediate walking potential. The physical therapist works to reinforce the teaching of the nurse.

In situations where the patient will never ambulate, wheelchair independence becomes all-important. The physical therapist may then assume a large part of the teaching and devote the patient's time in the department solely to these wheelchair activities since the nurses' time cannot be entirely spent on this phase of the program.

AMBULATION

The majority of inpatients have taken only a few assisted steps before they are admitted to a rehabilitation unit. Often, they have been entirely bedridden and when standing is attempted, they become dizzy, faint, and nauseated. This indicates the need for the standing or tilt table that gradually raises the patient from the supine to the standing position in degrees measured from 0 degrees to 90 degrees (see Fig. 80). On this device, supported by straps across the chest and knees, they are gradually accustomed to the upright position and eventually lose the unpleasant sensation when in vertical alignment. From day to day, the patient may progress either by increasing the amount of time spent at a certain angle or by increasing the size of the angle. Ideally, the patient is discontinued on the tilt table once he is able to stand twenty to thirty minutes at 80 to 90 degrees. As soon as the therapist

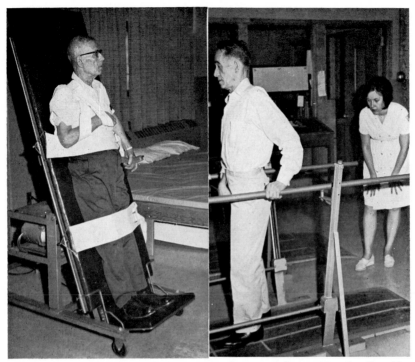

FIGURE 80 Patient becoming accustomed to upright position in tilt table.
FIGURE 81. Patient ambulating within security of parallel bars so therapist can stand off and analyze for gait pattern deficits.

feels that the patient has become accustomed to the upright position, standing is initiated in the parallel bars.

As soon as the patient begins standing and walking in the parallel bars it gives him a feeling of maximum support and allows the therapist to stand away and evaluate his gait (see Fig. 81). If a balance problem is noted, the therapist starts working on this, rather than allowing the patient to continue walking, establishing poor gait habits that will require correcting at a later date. The parallel bars also provide a good place to try assistive walking aids. Posterior splints will prevent the affected knee from flexing in the stance phase, and a dorsiflexor assist may minimize toe drag and prevent supination of the foot (see Chap. VI, Figs. 13-16 and Chap. VII, Figs. 28 and 29). Later, it may be necessary to order permanent orthetic devices to correct these deficits, but they may finally be discarded.

Once the patient has acquired some degree of skill in ambulation within the parallel bars, he is tried outside them. Again, assistive appliances are utilized as necessary to correct gait defects. Walking aids such as standard canes, Lofstrand crutches, or four-legged canes are employed at various levels of security. As the patient begins ambulating outside the bars, attempts are made to make him increasingly independent of the therapist. He may at first require a great deal of assistance, and this is gradually reduced to supervision. Then, if possible, supervision is withdrawn. An attempt is also made to reduce the number and complexity of walking aids.

As ambulation becomes functional as well as cosmetically improved, the therapist requests that the patient be ambulated on his ward. This may begin as short walks in the evenings and on weekends and progress to walking to and from the various therapy appointments that the patient has scheduled during the day. Simultaneously, as the patient's gait improves and his endurance increases, he spends less time in a wheelchair. Once he is safe on his feet, the chair is gradually taken from him in the morning, afternoon, then completely. This, of course, is the ideal situation with the patient that attains functional independence. Occasionally, when balance problems or poor judgment remain, the patient must utilize the wheelchair for safety's sake when alone and walk only with supervision.

If a stroke patient is ambulatory upon admission, his program is picked up at an advanced stage. The gait is evaluated for the following deficits and their degree of severity: loss of balance, hip drop, *genu recurvatum,* toe drag, supination of foot, hip adduction, knee flexion in stance phase, variance in stride, and weak push-off. Once these deficits are noted by the therapist, a suitable program is devised in order to correct as many as possible. Depending on the defect, balance exercises may be instituted, stretching or strengthening of certain muscle groups may be initiated, faulty habits may need correction by supervised ambulation, substitution of a motion by different muscle groups may be encouraged, or perhaps an orthetic device or walking aid prescribed.

At discharge, if the patient is to require equipment, the physical therapist assumes the task of ordering the proper devices agreed upon by the team. They must take into consideration the patients range of motion, the strength available to operate the device, the weight of the device, the amount of adjustment needed to operate the equipment, and the gadget tolerance of the patient. The equipment purchased must fulfill a definite need and may be required for safety, support, alignment, assistance, substitution, or movement. Other family and environmental factors must be considered such as the amount of money available for the device, where it is to be used, how much maintenance will be required, how much help is required by others for utilization, what the possibility is of adapting equipment already in the home, what the cost of the device is in relation to its usefulness, and whether it can be adequately stored.

The items most frequently ordered for ambulatory patients are short-leg braces, and standard and four-legged canes. The additional equipment most often requested for the patients by

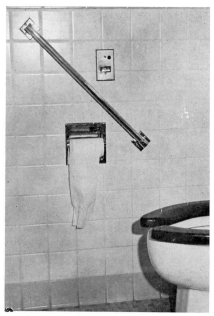

FIGURE 82. Wall grab bar next to toilet seat.

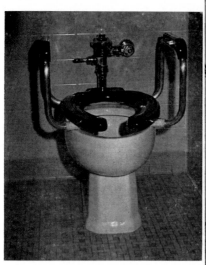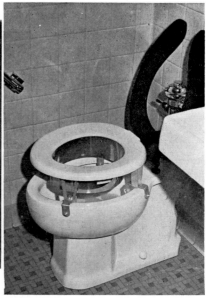

FIGURE 83.   Safety arms which are easily attached to most toilet bowls.
FIGURE 84.   Raised toilet seat.

physical therapists is in the area of activities of daily living. Tub
equipment includes guard rails that attach directly to the side
of the tub, bathtub seats for patients who experience difficulty
in transfer, and nonskid adhesive strips that are applied to the
tub bottom (see Chap. VII, Fig. 44). Toilet equipment includes
wall bars (see Fig. 82) or side rails attached to the seat (see
Fig. 83), and occasionally raised toilet seats (see Fig. 84).

In addition to the daily concentrated educational experience
provided for the patient, adequate attention and education must
be given to the family. The initial contact of family and therapist usually occurs when the relatives are asked to observe the
patient in the department. At that time, the therapist explains
the various types of exercise and equipment utilized and the
reasons for their use. At the same time, or at a later date (closer
to the patient's discharge) the family may be instructed in giving
the patient certain exercises and in how to assist or supervise in
ambulation, stairs, or transfer.

If a home visit is made prior to discharge, the family is again involved, for the therapist visits the home with the patient to answer questions, recommend practical changes within the home, and suggest equipment to enable the patient to perform as effectively as possible. If the therapist has had no prior contact with the family, he may take this opportunity to explain proper methods of transfer, guarding in ambulation, etc. (see Chap. XIV).

Without actual contact, the family may learn the purposes of the patient's activities in physical therapy through the family bulletin board that is located on the ward. This board is directed specifically to the family as an educational feature and is illustrated each month by a different rehabilitation service.

The physical therapist also assumes responsibility for the education of other professional and nonprofessional personnel. Many departments supervise junior and senior affiliating students from physical therapy schools within the area. Junior and senior affiliating nursing students are given introductory lectures on physical therapy and its relation to the nursing profession. Similar lectures are given to occupational therapy students.

Finally, the physical therapist is responsible for continuing his own education. This ranges from keeping up with current literature in the field, becoming involved in research projects and writing for publication, taking short-term courses and attending educational institutes, to participating actively in member organizations.

This chapter has concerned itself with the evaluation, treatment, and education of the stroke patient as they involve the physical therapist. Most specific methods employed in these three areas are commonly known. The author is aware that no one method is entirely right or wrong. Those discussed have been selected after much study and experience. It is the responsibility of the physical therapist to be aware of all treatment procedures and modalities applicable and to select those for each patient which will yield maximum results.

REFERENCES

BENNETT, R. L.: Functional testing and training in physical medicine. *Arch Phys Med*, 3:263, 1949.

DANIELS, L., WILLIAM, M., AND WORTHINGHAM, C.: *Muscle Testing, Techniques of Manual Examination*. Philadelphia, Saunders, 1956, pp. 1.6.

HOBERMAN, MORTON: Daily activity testing in physical medicine and rehabilitation. *Arch Phys Med, 33*:99, 1952.

HOLLIS, MARGARET, AND ROPER, MARGARET H. S.: *Suspension Therapy in Rehabilitation*. London, Bailliere, Tindall, and Cox, 1958, pp. 15-17.

KHALILI, A. A., AND BETTS, H. B.: Peripheral nerve block with phenol in the management of spasticity. *JAMA, 200*:1155, 1967.

KNOTT, M., AND VOSS, D. E.: *Proprioceptive Neuromuscular Facilitation: Patterns and Techniques*. New York, Hoeber, 1956, pp. 1-36.

LICHT, SIDNEY (Ed.): *Physical Medicine Library*, vol. 3, *Therapeutic Exercise*, 2nd ed. Baltimore, Waverly, 1961, pp. 296-306, 483, 731, and 774.

LYFORD, BERNICE, E., AND BONNER, CHARLES D.: An improvised method for sling suspension exercise. *Phys Ther Rev, 39*:530, 1959.

LYFORD, B. E.; BONNER, C. D., AND JOHNSON, M.: A new portable sling suspension apparatus. In Preparation.

MOORE, MARGARET L.: The measurement of joint motion: Part I: Introductory review of the literature. *Phys Ther Rev, 29*:195, 1949.

MOORE, MARGARET L.: The measurement of joint motion: Part II: The Technique of Goniometry. *Phys Ther Rev, 29*:256, 1949.

ROOD, M. S.: Neurophysiological mechanisms utilized in treatment of neuromuscular dysfunction. *Amer J Occup Ther, 10*:220, 1956.

SMITH, LAURA K.: Functional tests. *Phys Ther Rev, 34*:19, 1954.

Strike back at stroke. U. S. Dept. HEW, Public Health Service, U. S. Gov. Print., 1958, pp. 22-30.

TREANOR, W. J., AND REIFENSTEIN, G. H.: Potential reversibility of the hemiplegic posture. Results of reconstructive surgical procedure. *Amer J Cardiol, 7*:370, 1961.

WILLIAMS, MARIAN: Manual muscle testing, development, and current use. *Phys Ther Rev, 36*:797, 1956.

Chapter IX

ROLE OF THE OCCUPATIONAL THERAPIST

Of all team members, the occupational therapist is most universally misunderstood by physicians and by lay individuals. Because crafts are used in the pursuit of many goals, there is the mistaken impression that the patient is only being amused. He is being given something to do to occupy his time and mind.

Nothing can be further from the truth in a functional occupational therapy program. The contribution of this team member is vast, meaningful, and indispensible.

The patient who has had a stroke with resultant hemiparesis or hemiplegia is sent to occupational therapy by the physician to achieve one or more of the following treatment goals:

1. Functional use of the affected upper extremity.
   a. Increased strength and/or endurance.
   b. Improved range of motion.
   c. Improved coordination.
   d. Prevention of deformities.
2. General physical restoration.
   a. Increased sitting or standing tolerance.
   b. Improved work endurance.
3. Increased independence.
   a. Self-care activities.
   b. Other activities of daily living.
   c. Homemaking activities.
4. Prevocational assessment.
5. Maintain or improve mental health.

The usual referral form gives the patient's name, age, diagnosis, time since onset, medical complications, and hospital ward. In addition there may be a checklist of treatment goals such as that above, on which the solutions to the patient's probable problems are indicated in a very general manner. Occupational therapy evaluations are necessary to locate the exact problems, determine their severity and indicate which problems may be ameliorated by treatment. A complete assessment of the patient allows the therapist to plan the most effective treatment program. It also provides a complete picture of the patient against which progress can be measured.

ASSESSMENT OF THE PATIENT

Some of the rehabilitation problems commonly discovered by occupational therapy evaluations are discussed below along with the instruments used to reveal them.

Functional Use of Affected Upper Extremity

A variety of tools are available which measure the patient's ability to use his affected arm for purposeful activities. The tools selected should reveal enough information concerning the presence and/or severity of certain phenomena usually associated with hemiparesis or hemiplegia. This will influence prescription or prognosis in the perceptual motor area and will be discussed first.

Gross Limb Synergies

Synergies are primitive automatic movements which appear in the affected upper extremity when the patient attempts any voluntary movement of the arm or when he makes a major muscular effort in another part of his body. When synergies are dominant, they are the only motor response possible. If the patient tries to reach out to the table or down to his legs with the affected upper extremity, the only movement which will appear is one of two synergies. Which one appears depends upon the influence of the tonic neck reflex. Each of the two patterns can appear in its entirety, but more frequently the patient can perform only the stronger parts of the synergy. The flexion synergy, which consists of shoulder girdle elevation and adduction, shoulder abduction and external rotation, elbow flexion and forearm supination, may be present only in its strong elbow flexion component. The extension synergy consists of shoulder girdle abduction, shoulder internal rotation and adduction, elbow extension and forearm pronation. Again, only the strong shoulder internal rotation and adduction may appear.

Initially, synergies may be the only response a patient can make and later in his motor recovery they still might continue to influence purposeful movement. Careful observation and testing may discover that some muscles are able to contract only in certain movement patterns. The biceps brachii may contract strongly to flex the elbow, a part of the previous dominant flexion synergy, but not be able to contract to supinate the forearm. An adequate evaluation should discover if and in what manner the primitive synergies still influence patient's motor patterns.

Spasticity

Another factor impeding normal movement is spasticity. It not only interferes with the patient's free use of whatever strength the spastic muscle has but it prevents the free use of the antagonistic muscles. Because the spasticity pattern is determined by the patient's posture, the muscles influenced and the degree of influence should be assessed in both the upright and kneeling positions. When the patient is sitting or standing upright, spasticity is frequently present in the pectoralis major, biceps, pronator teres, and wrist, finger and thumb flexors. Gravity acting against weakened or paralysed muscles and the pull of these spastic muscles determine the patient's posture of shoulder girdle depression, shoulder inward rotation and adduction, elbow flexion, forearm pronation, and wrist, fingers and thumb flexion. When the patient assumes the quadrapedal position, the spasticity pattern usually changes, appearing in muscles which tend to support the patient in this position.

Sensation

Proprioceptive and cutaneous sensation are critical to movement, guiding its form, duration, and force. With diminished sensation, there is diminished spontaneous movement. Such movement which does take place does so under the continuous conscious control of the patient and is frequently suited only for gross tasks. So much of the energy of the patient can be used for conscious vigilance over movement that patients' become quickly fatigued. So much of their attention can be demanded by the movement that only a little is left over to give to the rest of their environment. The tasks which they are able to do are undemanding repetitive motor tasks. In addition there is some evidence that loss of or diminished sensation can contribute to psychological regression. Regression is a factor frequently complicating the rehabilitation of a CVA patient.

Coordination

It is necessary to discover not only if coordination has been affected, but also which of several factors might be affecting it. Some of the reasons for poor coordination are the influence of synergies, spasticity, and diminished or lost sensation. Any disorder of normal postural reflex mechanisms affects coordination. These equilibrium reactions and the adaptive changes in muscle tone which serve as a protection against the pull of gravity are basic to skilled voluntary movement. Another basic

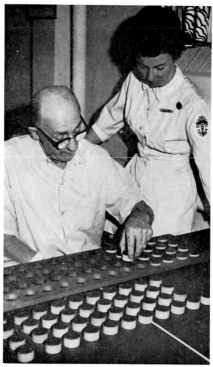

FIGURE 85. Patient performing Minnesota Rate of Manipulation Test with nondominant, nonaffected extremity as measure of gross coordination.

factor is the integrated use of both sides of the body. Many patients with no apparent residual of hemiparesis are unable to perform similar or alternating bilateral rhythmical tasks.

Gross and fine coordination can be evaluated on any test with acceptable validity and reliability. It is important that the test scores be considered cautiously. Many factors which have nothing to do with coordination can influence the patient's performance. A patient's lack of interest in performing well or his distractability or many other conditions can cause wide fluctuations in test results. Scores should be coupled with judgment to determine how well they reflect the ability of the patient (see Figs. 85-87).

Muscle Weakness

If the patient has isolated control of his upper extremity, that is, if he can independently move his shoulder, elbow, and hand, a manual muscle test may be of some value. Because occupational

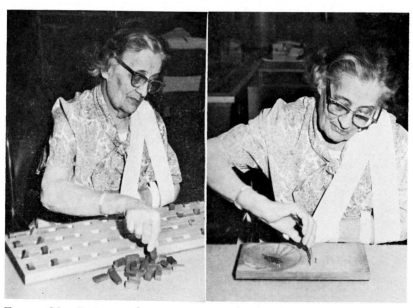

FIGURE 86. Patient performing gross test for coordination utilizing square instead of round pegs.

FIGURE 87. O'Connor Tweezer Test used to measure the patients ability for five-finger dexterity.

therapy is concerned with the patient's ability to do purposeful activities, the muscle test should be aimed at assessing the strength of functional muscle groups rather than that of individual muscles. The results of even so gross a test of strength should be viewed with caution, for any degree of spasticity or abnormal inhibition can interfere with the amount of force which a muscle group is actually able to exert. The test gives a picture of the amount of available force in functional muscle groups which can be exerted at least once when the patient is in the test position. This information has some value when it is placed with all the other information gathered about the patient and used with understanding.

Endurance

An assessment of endurance in the affected upper extremity is particularly important in two areas: the amount of time the scapula-shoulder unit can support the weight of the entire arm, and the amount of time the hand can perform fine coordinated tasks before spasticity and/or fatigue interferes with function. These two factors strongly influence the patient's functional use of the upper extremity. The scapula-shoulder unit is the mechanism which places and holds the hand in a position to work. Without strength and endurance in this unit, the hand has lost most of its value as a tool with which to explore and manipulate the physical environment. The hand itself frequently may have regained strength but repeated activity or the stress of a fine activity may cause such increased spasticity that function is lost soon after any activity is begun.

Range of Motion

A standard range of motion evaluation should be administered in order to gain a picture of the area within which the patient can move. The ranges of motion in the joints are usually limited by such conditions as severe spasticity and/or contractures. These conditions as well as any deformities should be noted. Information gained by this test is useful in determining solutions to problems in the ADL, homemaking, or vocational areas.

Spontaneous Use

A valuable part of the assessment of motor performance is the amount of use the patient makes of the available function in his arm. Close observation will reveal the degree to which the arm is used and the tasks for which it is used. The types of grasp pattern utilized when working should be compared to the types of grasp patterns which the patient can produce on demand. The patient may be using only primitive patterns even though more highly developed patterns are physically possible.

Visual perception impairment is a frequent residual of cerebral insult and may include homonymous hemianopsia, defects in perception of vertical and/or horizontal, disorientation in space, disturbance in body scheme or in form and size perception, and apraxia.

In establishing the precise long- and short-term occupational therapy objectives, designed to increase functional use of the affected upper extremity, the occupational therapist must be able to locate the exact problems, determine their severity, and judge their influence on successful rehabilitation too. Patients four months postinsult who have severe loss of sensation, who move only in limb synergies and make no spontaneous attempt to use the arm even as a paperweight, may have no occupational therapy goals aimed toward increasing functional use of their arm. The only proper goal involving the affected arm might be the amelioration or prevention of deformities through proper sling support and splinting. Patients one month postinsult who have intact sensation, have voluntary movement outside of synergies and who make attempts to use the limb in some tasks would probably have several long-term goals aimed at functional improvement of the upper extremity. The factors chosen for immediate treatment depend upon the judgment of the therapist which might well be based on his assessment of the patient in other areas.

Other Results of Cerebral Insult

The patient is more than a body with impaired function, and because cerebral insults can affect more than the patient's arm and legs, evaluation of the patient must extend into other areas than just the physical.

Cerebral insults always result in some permanent defect ranging in seriousness from being so minor that only results of exhausting testing compared to results of exhausting testing pre-insult would reveal their presence, down the scale to being so major they make rehabilitation an impossibility.

Homonymous Hemianopsia

A loss of one half of the visual field of each eye on the affected side is usually easily detected. If the condition is present its functional significance should be assessed. Patients who have such a loss may not spontaneously compensate for the loss or may even be unaware of the loss. These patients can leave uneaten all the food on the unseen part of their tray of food, leave unfinished all the work on their OT activity which is unseen, or walk into objects which are in the affected field of vision. On the other hand, some patients do turn their heads so as to see the environment toward their affected side. These behaviors should be noted in judging the extent to which homonymous hemianopsia may affect patient's safety and independence.

Difficulties in the Perception of Vertical and Horizontal

A rotation of the visual field is usually aggravated by poor lighting and may be one of the reasons for deteriorated functional performance in a darkened room, outside at night, or in a poorly lighted stairwell. Observation of patient's performance in these environments would lead to a more complete evaluation and knowledgable precautions.

Disorientations in Space

Problems in space perception and judgments with impairment of coordinated manipulation of the physical environment can be evaluated by the Ayres Space Test. If other complications prevent the valid use of this tool, clinical tests and judgments must be used as a basis for assessment.

Disturbance of Body Scheme

A frequent defect of patients who have cerebral lesions is body scheme disorientation. These patients may have difficulty in visualizing their bodies and how they are put together, or they may have difficulty recognizing left and right and in distinguishing between their fingers. Such difficulties can be detected by using clinical tests of body scheme. Defects in this area can affect the patient's coordination and/or his ability to perform self-care activities. For example, patients who are not aware of their affected side may not groom or dress that side of their bodies, despite the aid of mirrors or the prompting of the therapist (see Figs. 88 and 89).

Disorientation of Form and Size Perception

Patients who have disturbance in form and size perception tend to present mixed pictures of difficulties, being able to manipulate correctly the complex form of their clothing, but unable to put a square block in the correct place on a square and

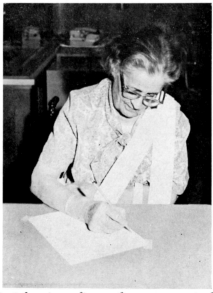

FIGURE 88. Patient drawing a figure of a man as part of body scheme test.

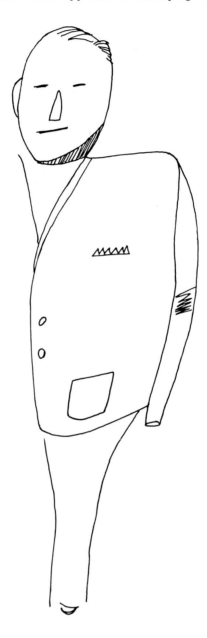

FIGURE 89.   Drawing of man done by a left hemiparetic. Note complete denial of left side of body.

circle cutout board. Form and size perceptual tests based on maturational development are useless as these patients present a picture of scattered developmental ability. Assessment must be done by observation of patient failures and successes.

Apraxia

This condition can seriously affect the patient's visual motor performance. Apraxia is the inability to perform desired activities not from any physical disability, but because of defects in ideation. Patients can move but do not know how to accomplish the desired goal. Simple clinical tests, such as asking the patient to pin a safety pin to a piece of cloth or paper can detect the presence of such defects. Many patients, realizing the difficulty they have in performing any purposive activity, prefer not to move at all. These patients are frequently thought by un-observant or overworked staff to be unmotivated. This error can only add to the great stress already being experienced by the patient.

General Physical Restoration

Occupational therapy is usually requested to increase the patient's sitting or standing tolerance and to improve work endurance. Evaluation of these areas is usually a matter of timing. The patient is given an activity which he is known to enjoy and the length of time he can work while comfortably seated or standing is noted. If work endurance is being evaluated, the data recorded should include the task being done by the patient and his rate of work so that some estimate can be made of the energy output during the work period.

Increased Independence

Certain cerebral insults can cause more problems than hemiplegia or hemiparesis. Some of the problems are so minimal that they display little noticeable effect on the rehabilitation process while others are so major they limit rehabilitation to the attainment of only minimal goals. They affect all treatment but present the greatest barrier to achieving independence. These problems can be determined in some cases by frank clinical procedures, but for the most part their discovery and assessment depend upon observation and interview techniques.

The ability of the therapist to note a variety of behaviors and to interpret them in light of his educated judgment makes observation one of the most important data gathering tools. The therapist's skill in using this technique depends upon his awareness of the effect these defects can have on behavior. Incidents which are illustrative of the influence of pathology should include the situation in which the incident took place and the exact verbal and nonverbal behavior of the patient and of pertinent other people. When sufficient incidents are gathered, possible causes for the behavior can be hypothesized.

Skilled interview techniques are especially important in gaining and understanding of the patient's attitudes and reactions, not only in the beginning of the treatment process, but throughout his rehabilitation. The occupational therapist is not limited to interviewing in an office, but may use the patient's daily treatment as a natural beginning point. Much valuable information can be gained from discussions among small groups of patients as they work (see Fig. 90).

Neurological problems which can be discovered by observation and interview and are basic to a patient's ability to relearn

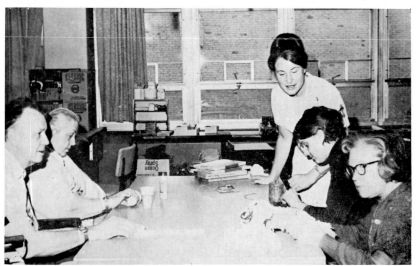

FIGURE 90. Small groups work together to foster interaction.

and maintain independence are (1) lower level of abstraction, (2) reduced retentiveness, and (3) reduced spontaneous motivation.

Lowered level of abstraction: When a patient has lost some of his ability to deal in abstractions, he frequently exhibits what is called poor judgment, that is, he is unable to think of what effects his present behavior will have on his future, future time being an abstraction. Patients with such a defect have learning problems. A patient may never lock his wheelchair before standing because he cannot project himself into the future so as to foresee the unstabilized wheelchair rolling back causing him to fall. The rule to lock the wheelchair before standing is therefore a rule without meaning or valid application to his behavior. Theories of learning describe how much more difficult it is to learn what seems to be without meaning.

Reduced retentiveness: Another problem with serious implications on rehabilitation success is poor memory. Material must be covered many times before the patient remembers it. Self-care activities, for example, may have to be presented as new each day for weeks before the patient remembers how to do them. Habit training over long periods of time may be the only way a patient learns and this limits how much he can learn. One method of evaluating retentiveness is through timed learning periods. The period it takes for a patient to learn a five-step activity the first time it is presented should be noted. The number of treatments the activity must be presented before the patient achieves independence in the activity should also be counted. The length of time a patient is able to concentrate on one activity without being distracted can also be timed to gain a picture of the patient's attention span.

Motivation: This one word has many meanings in rehabilitation. It usually refers to whether a cooperative patient progresses satisfactorily toward the rehabilitation goals which have been determined by his physical potentials. Satisfactory progress is usually the result of a consistent effort on the patient's part to achieve realistic goals within each of the rehabilitation disciplines. It requires a large daily output of energy to work satisfactorily every day in every area. Some patients do not seem to have the necessary energy. This lack makes difficult an accurate assessment of the capacities of the patient. It is easy to overestimate the severity of the patient's disability when the patient is not motivated to perform well. It is especially difficult to obtain the patient's maximum effort in tasks which present the greatest possibility of failure. Accurate evaluation is complicated by the fact that patients with serious defects in spontaneous motivation can present a clinical picture similar to that of a depressed patient who is passive and withdrawn. Very close observation of behavior during the period of trial treatment is needed before conclusions can be made about the real causes of the problem.

Evaluation and training in ADL activities is currently in a state of change. For years the occupational therapist was responsible for bringing the patient to independence in such activities as washing and grooming, dressing, and eating. Today many rehabilitation centers rely on rehabilitation nursing to perform this function. In these centers the occupational therapist acts as a consultant to the nursing staff and/or as a resource person when the patient needs special equipment and adapted devices or presents problems in areas basic to successful performance (see Figs. 91-94).

One area halfway between ADL and prevocational exploration is the retraining of the disabled housewife to independent function in as many homemaking tasks as possible. Whether the patient is to return to her own home or to be discharged to

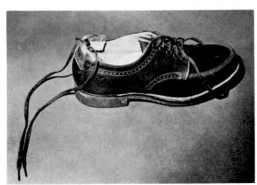

FIGURE 91.   Molded plastic shoehorn fitted to shoe. It is removed by pulling on strings.

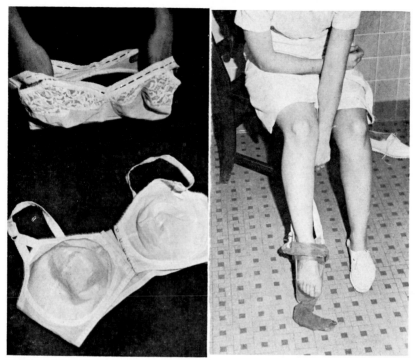

FIGURE 92. Elastic stretch and front fastening bras which facilitate independence in dressing.
FIGURE 93. Stocking aid which makes it possible to pull stocking over foot and up leg independently.

the home of a relative, an assessment and training for independence in some household tasks are usually necessary. The more independent the housewife becomes, the less the family must look to the community for assistance. Older women moving into the home of relatives usually feel and are less of a guest in the home and more an accepted family member if they have some recognized household duty. Although women are routinely assessed and retrained in household activities, men occasionally need some training. Disabled men who live alone or whose wives now work to help support the family frequently find it necessary to learn how to cook, clean, and shop.

There are several evaluative steps necessary before housekeeping retraining should be started. The first is a review of the

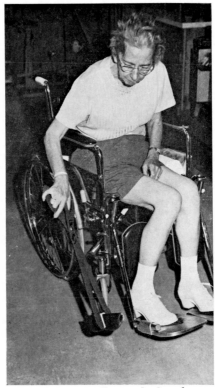

FIGURE 94. Tongs which are usually made by the patient as a project make it possible to reach for objects in difficult places.

patient's functional status with the prognosis for any future improvement. The second is an assessment of the environment in which the patient will be living after discharge. The third is an investigation of the patient's homemaker role and the rhythm of her work before the disability, along with an assessment of the patient's feelings about various household tasks. Fourth is an assessment usually from the social worker of the financial assets of the family and the amount of family support available after discharge. Finally the patient is asked to perform activities which he might be doing after discharge while the occupational therapist observes and notes his work method and any difficulties encountered (see Figs. 95-99).

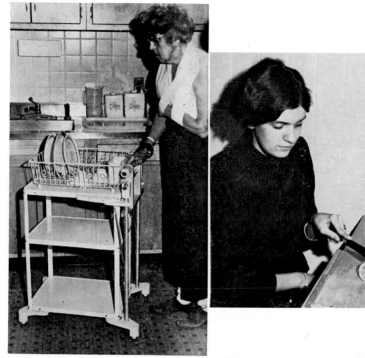

FIGURE 95.   Special utility cart designed by Mr. Harry E. Dow of Beverly, Mass., has gliders instead of wheels and a brake mechanism controlled by the nonaffected extremity at each step.

FIGURE 96.   Fruits or vegetables are impaled on two nails which are driven through a cutting board. This secures the item and permits one handed slicing or peeling of skins.

Prevocational Assessment

Occasionally patients who have had a cerebrovascular accident are candidates for reemployment. If they are still able to continue their former jobs and the job is available, there is little problem, but such a situation is rare. Most of the patients require vocational assessment and counseling. The occupational therapist is able to obtain and provide the vocational counselor with a great deal of information which he will find of use in quickly discovering the patients who may be major problems or who may be placed in appropriate jobs. Obtaining this informa-

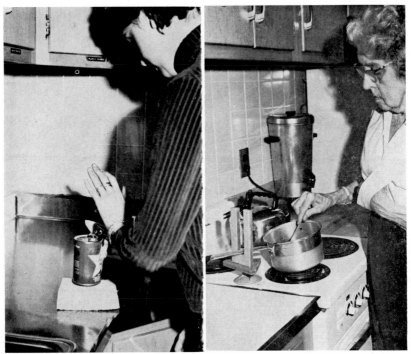

FIGURE 97.   One type of one-handed can opener.
FIGURE 99.   Suction stand for pot handle allows patient to stir while cooking
without the pot turning around.

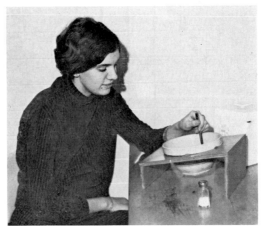

FIGURE 98.   Stand for mixing bowl which provides stability while stirring.

tion in occupational therapy is frequently called "prevocational evaluation" as if it were a single and separate evaluative procedure. It actually is not. Included in the prevocational evaluation should be all the information already gathered about the patient's perceptual motor ability and his level of independence in ADL. Of special importance in this latter situation is such information as the time it takes for the patient to perform blocks of activity. This includes time required to get up and prepare for the day, time required to eat lunch, and so forth. Also important is the notation of special equipment the patient needs for independence. If the patient needs reaching tongs in order to pick something up off the floor, this can be a factor to consider in successfully placing the patient in a job.

Also included in the prevocational assessment is a report on the patient's work habits. This includes such facts as the patient's punctuality, the neatness of his work, his independence in his work, how quickly he learns, the amount of supervision that is necessary, the length of time he can stay continuously at one activity, and so forth. Work habits are a critical factor in placement success and should be a major part of any prevocational evaluation.

A factor which can greatly influence placement success is the patient's ability to get along with others, both those in authority and his peer group. The patient's ability to begin and maintain successful interpersonal relationships can be carefully observed by the occupational therapist.

Finally the vocational counselor is interested in the attitudes the patient has displayed in occupational therapy. He is especially interested in the patient's attitude toward various types of work, toward wage earning in general, and in the patient's expectations about his work future. Many patients who have been employed in jobs with high pay and high status may reject the idea of working for less money or at a job with less social status, even though they seem to recognize their inability to perform as well as they did formerly. The vocational counselor can assist them make this long and difficult adjustment and it saves time if the vocational counselor has an awareness of this problem as early in the rehabilitation process as possible.

If available, job samples in major appropriate job families may be administered to the patient to define the patient's abilities. Job samples such as those used in the Tower system should be supplemented whenever possible with job trial periods so the occupational therapist can judge not only how well the patient does in a job which is new, but how he can function on a job over a period of time such as one to four weeks. Such pre-vocational procedures are valuable predictors of job success in specific job families. As time-consuming as they are, they can be time-savers as they allow the vocational counselor to place the patient in a job which he is known to perform well and which he is known to enjoy.

Certain evaluations should be repeated every month so that success or failure of treatment can be noted and new treatment objectives introduced when appropriate. Evaluation of the functional ability in the affected upper extremity is one such procedure. Other evaluations are part of a continuous assessment process and continue during every treatment until discharge. An example would be the observation of patients' interaction with others. A few evaluations should be given only after a period of treatment has made possible a tentative judgment about the degree of rehabilitation the patient will achieve. For example, a job sample assessment should be started only when the patient's probably discharge status would make holding a job possible.

Mental Health

The most generally used evaluative procedures are interviews and observation. The usual problems encountered are depression, confusion, and distress caused by emotional lability and other conditions which interfere with the patient's successful interaction with others.

Depression

Depression usually has a solid basis in reality. The majority of patients who suffer CVA's are older people who are living through a period when they must adjust to the increasing autonomy of their children, to the possible loss of the marital partner, and to their retirement with the concomitant loss of status as a productive worker. Added to these possible stresses is the sudden and devastating loss of or impairment of function on one side of their bodies. Unfortunately, disability is looked at with distaste by most Americans, as they have had strong cultural training to give high value to a young and unimpaired body. Now these patients, many of whom are making the difficult adjustment to the process of aging, find themselves with a crippled body. Many patients have strong sense of rejection. Not only do they reject their own newly disabled bodies, but many find that they are being rejected by their families who fear the burden of a disabled person in the home or who merely feel that their home has no place for an older grandparent. The discovery of the exact dynamics of a patient's depression and their manipulation for the recovery of mental health belongs to psychiatric, psychological, and social service team members. But as long as the patient is one person, every rehabilitation discipline can and should contribute to the mutual understanding of the patient and to the treatment of his depression.

Emotional Lability

Emotional lability in which the patient is easily moved to tears sometimes by inappropriate stimulii should be noted because it frequently is a cue that the patient is at that moment undergoing a stressful situation. It might be that the patient is new to the environment and under the stress of learning his new role and of locating new sources of psychological support. It might be that the demands the therapist is making upon the patient are too great, and the therapist should cut them back to within the patient's tolerance. In any case emotional lability can be distressing to the patient who is embarrassed about crying frequently without a serious reason to justify such behavior, and also for the staff and other patients who have been taught by our culture that only under the most serious stress, which automatically demands great sympathy from all, will anyone cry. The staff must be able to deal with their own uneasiness towards a patient's emotional behavior without reacting hostilely to the patient for causing such unease. The patient-therapist relationship is important in assisting the patient to make his maximum gains. Any factor which can upset this relationship must be discovered and the cause understood. The staff must also be able to explain the emotional lability to other patients so that there is acceptance of the patient in his own peer group.

Confusion

Many patients experience confusion for varying lengths of time after their cerebral insult, especially at night. The confusion may be exacerbated after the transfer of the patient to a rehabilitation center and only subside after the patient becomes familiar with his new environment or after correction of any physical cause. If periods of confusion are noted, evaluative procedures which require the patient's best performance should be delayed until the patient is fully oriented or until the therapist becomes skilled in noting periods of bewilderment. Other patients can be helped to understand the occasional disturbing behavior of the confused patient in an effort to obtain group acceptance.

OCCUPATIONAL THERAPY TREATMENT

Once the thorough evaluation in occupational therapy has been completed, the patient's specific problems are outlined along with a judgment as to their vulnerability to treatment. Staff conferences with other disciplines assist in deciding which problems will be attacked in the first treatment program. The exact treatment to assist the restoration of function in the affected body parts and the restoration of correct perception cannot be discussed as they vary widely depending on the theoretical beliefs and the experience of each therapist. Undoubtedly, in some distance future, research will prove some theories and procedures superior to others in effecting maximum return of function, but at the present time therapists use treatment procedures which they think are most adequately supported by past research and/or which they have found to be most successful in their own clinical experience.

Treatment procedures in some areas can be discussed, however, in order to give a basic understanding of the application of occupational therapy. When a patient has little to no probability of regaining function in the affected upper extremity the usual goals of therapy are to (1) prevent deformities in the affected arm, (2) increase skill in use of the unaffected hand, (3) maintain mental health, and (4) assist in regaining independence. The attainment of these goals will be discussed below.

Prevention of Deformities

The usual deformities developing from paralysis and/or spasticity in the upper extremity have been discussed in other chapters. The occupational therapist participates as much as

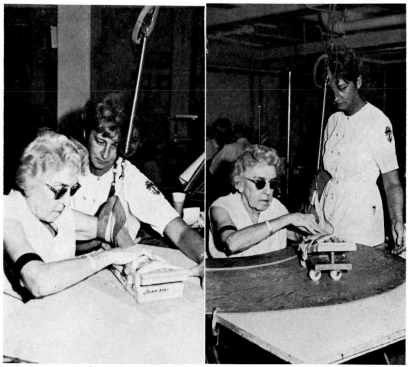

FIGURE 100. Sling suspension allows patient to put paralyzed extremity through passive range of motion while sanding wood. The nonaffected extremity provides the motor power for the affected extremity to which sanding block is strapped.

FIGURE 101. Skateboard permits active exercise of a weak upper extremity in adduction and abduction. Friction has been minimized.

possible in these three areas: range of motion, proper positioning, and adequate splinting. Passive range of motion of an
affected extremity may be done several times during the occupational therapy treatment period. Certain motions of the upper
extremity are performed passively by the patient himself by
using his unaffected arm to move the affected one in an activity
such as sanding (see Figs. 100 and 101). The occupational
therapist must also see to it that the patient is properly positioned
while under his supervision. The spastic upper extremity is
placed on the wheelchair armboard, or in the outrigger sling
when sitting. If the upper extremity is faccid and the patient
is standing, the arm is placed in an over-the-head sling (see
Chapt. VI, Figs. 4-8 and 11-13).

Perhaps the greatest contribution is in the fabricating of
static splints. Although most occupational therapists make it

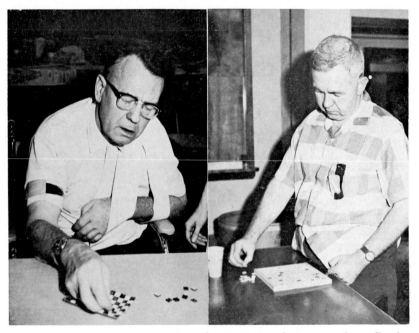

FIGURE 102. A project requiring the accurate placement of small tiles
fosters improvement in finger dexterity.
FIGURE 103 Working on projects in the upright position increases standing
tolerance and endurance.

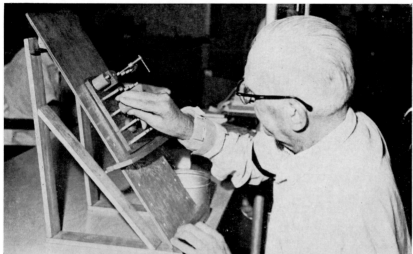

FIGURE 104. The placement of beads on pegs in an above shoulder activity helps to promote better coordination in shoulder and hand patterns.

clear that this responsibility is theirs by default, there are obviously too few orthetists available. Static splints are usually made to prevent deformities of fingers, thumb, and wrist. They should be lightweight, durable, washable, and fitted to each patient. The patient should be able to put it on and take it off without assistance (see Chap. VI, Figs. 19-21). Dynamic splints are at times assembled from commercially available kits. If an orthetist is available, occupational therapy should be concerned only with checking the fit or if the splint is dynamic in teaching the patient correct efficient usage.

Increase Skill in the Use of the Unaffected Arm

Clumsy use of the unaffected arm even in one-handed activities can be the result of perceptual problems such as spatial disorientation or apraxia. In many cases, however, where the problems are not so complicated, patients can be helped to develop skill in using one hand in their daily activities (see Figs. 102-104).

ADL tasks which need a high degree of dexterity should be practiced until they can be accomplished quickly with minimum energy. Examples of these activities are putting hair up in pin curls, putting on brace and shoe, getting change out of a wallet

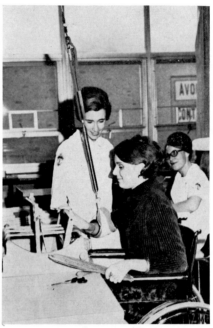

FIGURE 105. Sling suspension, by neutralizing gravity, allows a weak affected extremity to be used in an assisting capacity.

or pocketbook, and opening an envelope. The patient can be helped to be independent in many other activities by teaching general solutions to a variety of problems. To illustrate, generally in normal motor tasks one hand is used for manipulation while the other is used for stabilization. In hemiparetics, the unaffected hand can still manipulate but some other method of stabilization must be substituted for the nonfunctional hand. The substitution can be a C-clamp, the weight of the arm or trunk, a clothespin, the pinch of a partly closed drawer and so on (see Fig. 105). Patients are taught creative problem solving so they are better prepared for continued independence.

Maintain Mental Health

Most patients have rehabilitation programs which last from two to three months. During this time they must work hard toward goals that seem very distant. For instance, everyday they go to physical therapy to work toward independent ambulation and/or to speech to work toward improved ability to communicate. Progress frequently is slow and to the patients, it even can seem nonexistent. If every discipline demanded continuous wholehearted effort in working toward distant and seemingly unattainable goals, the patients might rapidly sink into a discouraged lethargy which would make all staff effort and skill unavailing. Patients need some experience at attaining concrete successes early in their rehabilitation program. In addition they need some experiences which demonstrate that their new bodies can be used to produce an acceptable product even if they regain no function in the affected upper extremity. One purpose of occupational therapy is to assist the patient in adjusting to his permanent disability by giving him the opportunity to discover that his body can still function successfully in doing whatever available activity he chooses to undertake. The standard for success in each activity is set by the patient rather than by the therapist or any master craftsman volunteer. The patient himself must think his product is praiseworthy.

In the beginning of the treatment program, some patients need to complete one object a day, but as the patient begins his adjustment and/or as he begins to see definite gains in other disciplines, he usually is able to undertake long-range activities. In occupational therapy the focus of his attention can remain on the objects he is making rather than on gains in endurance, range of motion, or coordination. So much prominence is given to the physical function of his body in rehabilitation that it may be therapeutic to put emphasis on what the patient is doing with his physical function rather than on how he physically functions. After all, in most cases there is some permanent residual loss which will prevent the patient's body from ever being "normal" again. Therefore one should not continuously emphasize how nearly normal he is when he may never reach the goal of being completely normal again. Occupational therapy emphasizes how effectively the patient is performing activities with his remaining physical abilities.

Assist in Regaining Independence

This goal and the goal of mental health can be discussed as

one in some areas. Almost every patient can be trained to have some degree of independence during his hospital stay. But unless the patient really wishes to be independent, he will rapidly become dependent again after discharge. Many factors contribute to a patient's dependence such as the cultural acceptance of an adult's abrogation of his responsibilities during illness and the belief that the sick role is a passive role in which the patient relies on the activities of others for his care and his comfort. The latter factor is reinforced by the acute hospital in which patients are usually washed, fed, and kept in swaddling clothes. During this acute hospital stay, patients may not have to make a single decision. They are told when to wake up, what they are to do, what they will eat, and so forth. Many patients learn quickly and permanently that their disability gains for them the passive dependent role of a child not only with the hospital staff, but also with their families. Their transfer to a rehabilitation unit can be an unwelcome shock as rehabilitation demands their active physical participation. It should, in addition, allow opportunities for the patient to begin acting like an independent adult who is able to make decisions and accept responsibilities. Patients can be given their appointment for occupational therapy and the responsibility of reporting on time. They can be encouraged to select one of several possible activities which would be of benefit to them. They can be expected to assist other patients, take out and put away their own tools and equipment, and so forth. In many ways they should be given the opportunity to relearn the enjoyment of being a responsible independent adult. When a patient wants to be independent he will find ways of becoming and remaining as independent as possible.

From the first interview to the last treatment the therapist should be aware of what the patient's rehabilitation goals are, what postdischarge lifestyle expectations he has, and what attitudes he has toward his disability. As the patient is encouraged to talk about these things, the therapist is made aware of problems which could, unless changed, prevent the patient from maintaining the independence which his physical capacity and training enable him to achieve. The occupational therapist along with every other profession should be concerned with helping the patient desire an active independent life. The occupational therapist not only teaches the patient the techniques of independence and provides the necessary equipment, but he also helps to carry out one or more of the following processes:

1. Helps the patient to emotionally accept and adjust to his physical handicap.

2. Provides emotional support and reassurance, especially when progress seems slow.

3. Instills realistic confidence in the future. This is of great value in motivating the patient to work diligently in treatment.

4. Provides the patient with an opportunity for free discussion of his feelings and problems, especially after home visits.

5. Prepares the patient for problems which may come up after discharge and discusses possible reactions, adjustments, and/or solutions.

6. Helps the patient realize that only part of his rehabilitation takes place in the rehabilitation setting. The rest of it takes place in his own home, and for the most part is his responsibility.

Unless the therapist skillfully uses the techniques of the counseling process, he will not achieve the desired goal of patient independence very frequently. The more skillful the therapist, and the more aware of psychodynamics the entire rehabilitation staff is, the more successfully will the hemiplegic patient be treated.

It should be noted that specific treatment methods have not been discussed. The tools of the occupational therapist are many and varied. They include crafts such as woodworking, ceramics, printing, weaving, metal work, sewing, painting, etc. Standard recreational work and homemaker activities are also used. The activity which is chosen to assist in achieving a specific goal depends upon the therapist's past experience and beliefs. In specific instances any one may be used. In daily practice each department has its favorites. Woodworking is widely used by the authors as it permits most occupational therapy goals of range of motion, increased strength, greater endurance, improved coordination, etc., to be attained, plus providing a useful end product for the patient to admire (see Fig. 106).

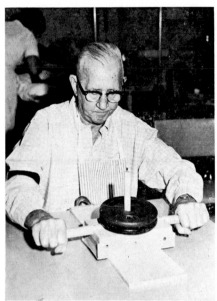

Figure 106.   Resistive exercise is provided by the use of a weighted sanding block.

REFERENCES

Ayres, A. J.: Occupational thearpy directed toward neuromuscular integration. In *Occupational Therapy*, edited by Willard and Spackman. Philadelphia, Lippincott, 1963.

Baker, R. G., et al.: *Adjustment to Physical Handicap and Illness*. New York, Soc. Sci. Res. Council, 1953.

Benton, A. L., and Fogel, M.: Three dimensional constructional praxis. *Arch Neurol*, 7:347, 1962.

Brunnstrom, S.: Motor behavior of adult hemiplegic patient. *Amer J Occup Ther*, 15:6, 1961.

Carroll, Virginia B.: Implications of measured visuospatial impairment in a group of left hemiplegic patients. *Arch Phys Med*, 39:11, 1958.

Delecato, G. H., and Doman, G.: Hemiplegia and concomitant psychological phenomena. *Amer J Occup Ther*, 11:186, 1957.

Gellhorm, E.: Patterns of muscular activity in man. *Arch Phys Med*, 28:568, 1947.

Goldstein, K.: *Aftereffects of Brain Injuries in War*. New York, Grune, 1942.

Gooddy, W.: Sensation and volition. *Brain*, 72:312, 1949.

Lashley, K. S.: Factors limiting recovery after cerebral nervous lesions. *J Nerv Ment Dis*, 88:733, 1938.

MacDonald, J.: An investigation of body scheme in adults with cerebral vascular accidents. *Amer J Occup Ther, 14*:75, 1960.

Reynolds, G. S., and Brunnstrom, S.: Problems of Sensorimotor Learning in the evaluation and treatment of the adult hemiplegic patient. *Rehab Lit, 20*:163, 1959.

Ruch, T. C.; Fulton, J. F., and German, W. J.: Sensory discrimination in monkey, chimpanzee, and man after lesions of parietal lobe. *Arch Neurol Psychiat, 34*:919, 1938.

Third International Congress, World Federation of Occupational Therapists, 1962. Study Course III, Dynamic Living for the Long Term Patient. Dubuque, W. C. Brown, 1964.

Third International Congress, World Federation of Occupational Therapists, 1962. Study Course VI, Approaches to the Treatment of Patients With Neuromuscular Dysfunction. Dubuque, W. C. Brown, 1964.

Twitchell, T. E.: The prognosis of motor recovery in hemiplegia. *Bull Tufts-New Eng Med Cent, 3*:146, 1957.

Twitchell, T. E.: The restoration of motor function following hemiplegia in man. *Brain, 74*:443, 1951.

Van Buskirk, C., and Webster, D.: Prognostic value of sensory defect in rehabilitation of hemiplegics. *Neurology, 5*:407, 1955.

Chapter X

ROLE OF THE SPEECH THERAPIST

THE SPEECH THERAPIST is a valuable team member for those stroke patients with communication problems. Speech difficulties after a stroke often manifest themselves as partial or complete loss of the ability to speak or to comprehend the spoken word. In broader terms, this problem, *aphasia,* may be defined as a loss of symbolic formulation and/or expression due to a brain lesion.

Another speech difficulty, *dysarthria,* a disorder of articulation due to impairment of that portion of the central nervous system which directly controls the muscles of articulation, may also occur. This results in sluggish or slurred speech due to an actual inability to move the articulators correctly. In aphasia, however, the speech mechanism may be unaffected, but the patient's language appears to be garbled, disconnected, halting, or almost nonexistent. It has been said that aphasia in most instances manifests itself as *abnormal* language rather than as total absence of speech.

It is the aim of the speech therapist to help the patient attain the highest level of communication of which he is capable. Better communication between staff and patient is also sought. The patient must want to communicate and must feel that his efforts are accepted and not derided. The problem of frustration will be discussed later, but it should be stated that the patient who accepts the notion that he is not expected to speak and that his efforts at conveying thoughts are not given attention will not speak.

It is therefore the speech therapist's responsibility to provide the aphasic patient with instruction in communication to the extent that the patient can indicate his needs as intelligibly as possible. The speech therapist aids the patient in understanding simple verbal orders so that he becomes accustomed to the hospital routine. The therapist also explains the patient's level of communication to the staff and to his family so that they can understand the patient and be understood by him with as little difficulty as possible.

The tasks of the speech therapist have been outlined as follows: (1) to discover the linquistic potential remaining in the patient, (2) to evaluate this potential in terms of his reeducation in speech, and (3) to use this residuum most efficiently in speech therapy adapted to the individual.

SPEECH EVALUATION
Problems of Aphasia

Avoiding a Misdiagnosis

There are two common errors often made by beginning physicians in diagnosing aphasia. The first concerns the patient who does not speak at all. Such a patient either has other lesions of the nervous system or suffers from a psychiatric disorder. Aphasics are rarely speechless and can nearly always produce a few words.

The second type of patient is the severely dysarthric patient, particularly the one with bilateral cerebral lesions who presents the syndrome of pseudobulbar dysarthria. His speech may be incomprehensible and may lead the doctor to misdiagnose the case as aphasia, especially if other cerebral pathology is seen. The doctor must be able to ensure that the *language* of the patient is abnormal before labeling it as aphasia.

Localization of Brain Damage

The questions are frequently asked whether there is a need to know the area of the brain which has been damaged and what relationships may be found between the locus of the lesion and any abnormal language pattern.

The speech therapist does need to know the general medical condition of the patient and the doctor's judgment as to whether the condition is static or progressive. Simon stated that information on the locus of the lesion is of no value to a speech therapist. However, most therapists are interested in knowing the possible sites of lesions although they are more concerned with the presented abnormalities. It does seem defensible that some knowledge of the language areas of the brain would help in diagnosis, therapy, and prognosis.

It is the function of the examining physician to determine first whether aphasia exists. Aphasia must be established as distinct from other subcortical injuries such as blindness, deafness, and paralysis. It must also be distinguished from functional disturbances such as stuttering or hysterical aphonia. Second, the physician attempts to determine the nature and extent of cortical damage, because of the numerous possible areas which may have caused the malfunction. Third, it should be determined whether the lesion is unilateral, suggesting an undamaged area available for retraining. This can be done by assessing such signs as unilateral weakness of extremities, facial paralysis, a positive Babinski, or an homonymous hemianopsia on the side opposite the weakness.

Geschwind presents a scheme for localizing the lesions which have affected the patient's speech. Aphasias of the *fluent* variety (where speech retains the correct rhythm and melody and yet is empty of content) occur only with posterior lesions, that is, behind the Rolandic fissure, involving either the lower parietal or posterior temporal lobe. These lesions are posterior to the motor cortex and most patients have no hemiplegia.

Anterior lesions (in Broca's area) always produce *nonfluent* aphasias (an incapacity to utter long, grammatical utterances, but an ability to utter some language which is usually meaningful in context).

Some patients with posterior lesions may also be nonfluent. If the patient presents a nonfluent aphasia with hemiplegia, this indicates a lesion of Broca's area and the adjacent motor cortex. If the patient is nonfluent with little or no hemiparesis, he usually has a lesion of the posterior speech regions.

When the records of 1,166 brain-injured patients, most of whom were wounded during World War II by exploding missile fragments, were investigated, injuries producing aphasia occurred in the lower half of the precentral and postcentral gyrus, the supramarginal and the angular gyrus, the inferior parietal gyrus, and much of the temporal lobe according to Russel and Espir.

However, another study of young aphasics done by Eisenson (1947) found no reliable correlation between the type of language dysfunction and the site of the brain injury. The only consistent finding was that if the aphasic disturbances were still present three to four months after the incident of trauma, the injured area involved part of the contralateral brain hemisphere. The patients also showed no consistent relationship between the extent of their brain damage and their capacity to relearn language except where the amount of brain injury was extremely great and involved both hemispheres. It is also of interest that 95 per cent of the right-handed aphasic patients and 63 per cent of the left-handed and ambidextrous subjects in one survey done by Schuell, Jenkins and Jiménez-Pabón had left hemispheric lesions.

Tests Commonly Used

Various formal tests may be used to record the patient's level of response at a certain point or points in time. These tests are divided into portions covering the range of language functions. Tests are arranged differently but each should cover the areas of understanding the spoken word, understanding the written word, using the speech mechanism, using meaningful language, and writing. Each portion usually has several questions, testing from the simple to the complex. Some tests sample certain nonlanguage behavior to detect agnosias (failures to recognize and comprehend sensory stimuli although sensation is intact) and apraxias (inabilities to execute simple voluntary acts in the absence of paralysis).

The second use of these tests is to facilitate comparison of data between patients. A common test must be agreed upon if their performance is to be compared.

Any test must take into account the premorbid intelligence and education of the patient. It is ridiculous to ask the patient something to which he never knew the answer. For instance, one test asks "What is the capitol of New Hampshire?" Many nonaphasics cannot answer this question.

Tests should be presented objectively to the patient. The tester should explain that he is trying to find the language areas which are causing trouble, that some of the questions may be easy and others will be difficult. No false approval of incorrect responses is necessary since the patient is aware that the troublesome areas will be noted for further work.

Two widely used tests are Eisenson's Examining for Aphasia (1954) and the Halsted, Wepman Screening Test for Aphasia (1949). Both provide a sampling of the patient's performance for the various language modalities. Both are fairly brief and will give an outline of the patient's abilities.

In response to requests for a short test for aphasia which would yield information about patterns of disability and prognosis, Schuell (1966) selected items from her Minnesota Test for Differential Diagnosis of Aphasia (1965). Tests scaled for difficulty permit the examiner to select an appropriate range of tests for each patient. In addition, a diagnostic scale and a severity scale are presented. These permit comparison of diagnostic patterns and severity of functional deficits across the range of modalities and over periods of time.

Language Modalities Test for Aphasia developed by Wepman and Jones (1961) provides another useful standardized test. Stimuli are presented by filmstrips in five response categories. The test is available in two equivalent forms, the initial items of both constituting a "screening section."

Taylor (1964b) distinguishes between functional communication and the patient's clinical performance. The patient's natural use of language (his functional ability) may differ widely from his performance on test materials. She devised a functional communcation profile which consists of fifty communication behaviors which occur in everyday situations. On the basis of informal interaction with the patient, the examiner rates what functional use the patient makes of his residual language.

Classification Systems

Aphasia is primarily a language deficit which affects various language modalities. Several classification systems have been devised to explore the range and severity of this deficit.

Many older schema were based on the dichotomy of motor and sensory categories and the concept of isolated pure disorders. The division between receptive and expressive aphasia has often been employed with varying terminology: input and output, decoding and encoding, passive and active evaluation and production. The problem lies less in the terminology used than in the fact that many examiners assume that everyone defines the terms as they do. In reality, there are almost as many diverging definitions as there are clinicians.

Wepman (1962) describes five types of language disturbances:

1. Global—a complete inability to comprehend or function with language symbols.

2. Jargon—an inability to produce meaningful speech.

3. Pragmatic—an inability to produce words which relate to the stimulus. Words which are produced are meaningless in context.

4. Semantic—an inability to use substantive speech. Speech efforts consist of connective words, have little meaning.

5. Syntactic—Absence of syntax or grammar but speech is meaningful, composed mostly of nouns, verbs, and modifiers with few or no connectives.

Schuell, Jenkins, and Jiménez-Pabón (1964) offer five diagnostic categories.

Group 1. Simple aphasia with reduction of available language in all modalities in the absence of specific perceptual, sensorimotor, or dysarthric components.

Group 2. Aphasia complicated by central involvement of visual processes.

Group 3. Aphasia with severe reduction of all language modalities complicated by sensorineural involvement.

Group 4. Aphasia with some residual language preserved and scattered findings that usually include both visual involvement and dysarthria.

Group 5. An irreversible aphasic syndrome characterized by almost complete loss of functional language skills.

The problem still remains that any classification system is difficult to apply to any particular patient. Most investigators agree, however, that no patient with "pure" aphasic symptoms exists.

Observations Concerning Patients with Nonlanguage Problems

Along with impairment of language there are many deviations

of a nonverbal nature. Wepman (1951) lists thirty-four such deviations:

1. Loss of attention and concentration.
2. Loss of memory.
3. Reduced association of ideas.
4. Abstract-concrete imbalance (loss of ability to abstract: concrete concept formation).
5. Poor organizing ability.
6. Poor judgment.
7. Perseveration.
8. Constriction of thought and interest.
9. Reduced ability to generalize, categorize, group, or plan future action.
10. Reduced general level of intelligence.
11. Reduced ability to inhibit internal emotional forces which disturb the action of the intellect (Halstead's "power factor").
12. Inability to shift.
13. Psychomotor retardation.
14. Feelings of inadequacy.
15. Egocentricity.
16. Increased irritability and fatigability.
17. Euphoria.
18. Social withdrawal and seclusiveness.
19. Reduced ability to adjust to new situations.
20. Catastrophic reactions.
21. Reduced initiative.
22. Disinterest in the environment, both physical and human.
23. Externalization of behavior; a lack of introspection or self-criticism.
24. Reduced spontaneity.
25. Perplexity (a distrust of one's own ability).
26. Automatic verbalization.
27. Impulsive behavior.
28. Regressive, infantile behavior.
29. Impotence (the inability to correct behavior one knows is wrong).
30. Post traumatic psychotic behavior showing illusions, hallucinations, delusions, and extravagant behavior.
31. Anxiety and tension.
32. Convulsive seizures.
33. Changing personality profile, the emergence and submergence of characteristics.
34. Hemiplegia.

The individuality of these symptoms must be stressed.

When first observing the patient, his responses to language should be noted. He may be unable to comprehend language as a meaningful form of communication. He may be able to follow simple one-step commands (touch your nose), yet be unable to perform more complex commands adequately (close your eyes and touch your nose with your finger).

The patient's attention span may be so short that he is unable to follow a command, or he may be experiencing pain which takes his attention away from verbal commands.

The patient's ability to change from one activity (or word) to another must be noted. Does he continue to use a previously correct response when it is no longer appropriate (perseveration)?

The patient's emotional tone must also be assessed. Is he labile? Does he overreact to stimuli? Does he swear or use other inappropriate language? Does he seem depressed? Euphoric? Hostile?

If the patient begins to laugh or cry excessively, this behavior should be accepted calmly and should be explained as being a common problem. This often will relieve male patients who are extremely embarrassed by their crying. If the patient seems unable to stop, some change of conversational topic, or perhaps a joke will help him break the perseverative response.

Depression is a realistic response to a loss; it indicates insight and a realization of the present situation. Euphoria is another possible reaction but may often be a denial of reality rather than a grieving acceptance of it. If the patient thinks he has no problems, he will be less apt to improve them since to him they are nonexistent or unimportant.

Does the patient say or indicate that he wants to get better, or does he accept the present situation without any apparent realization of his predicament?

Can he tolerate frustration or does he react catastrophically to pressure? Goldstein (1942) described catastrophic reactions as responses that are disordered, inconsistent, and inadequate. This behavior occurs when the patient cannot meet the demands placed upon him. Such situations should of course be avoided.

Investigating Language Modalities

Two questions should guide one in evaluating the patient's

aphasic deficits: To what extent is the patient's use of language reduced? What other specific deficits are present which may complicate the problem, such as impaired sensorimotor coordination, reduced discrimination of visual, auditory, or proprioceptive stimuli, disorientation in time or space, or dysarthria?

Auditory Comprehension

Just as most human communication depends primarily on the spoken word to impart meaning, so comprehension of oral speech is the major pathway for understanding others.

Results of one study by Schuell (1953) of 130 aphasic patients showed that all of them had some impairment in auditory reception. Investigation of this area is most important since the patient who seems unable to comprehend oral speech will most often be rejected by a rehabilitation unit if it is felt that he cannot understand verbal commands. Many patients who upon evaluation seem withdrawn, lethargic, or dull tend to respond adequately as they become accustomed to a regular routine. Some patients can follow verbal commands more easily if they are accompanied by gesture or demonstration, and often show physical recovery long before they are able to understand all of what is being said to them.

In testing the area of auditory comprehension, it is first necessary to ascertain whether the patient can actually hear what is being said to him. Since some hospitals remove patients' hearing aids upon admission because they are considered as valuables, the patient may be unable to understand what is going on around him. When the hearing aid is replaced after several weeks or months, the patient often must become reaccustomed to amplified stimulation. Such a patient then faces a double handicap: first, he must now readjust to oral communication from which he has been isolated; and second, he must adjust to a new situation in which his own speech may have been affected.

All but the most involved patients can be conditioned to respond to pure-tone audiometric testing. If hearing problems are suspected and an audiometer is not immediately available, tuning fork tests *for the speech frequencies* may be used (500, 1000, 2000 Hz). The patient will usually be able to indicate that

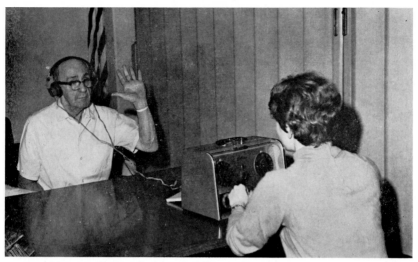

FIGURE 107. Hearing is an important part of communication. Testing is done with audiometer.

he senses the vibrations of the tuning fork. This method is limited, however, since the actual decibel level of the tuning fork is not known. Audiometric testing is recommended for all patients in the geriatric age group (see Fig. 107).

In evaluating the patient's auditory comprehension, an attempt is made to find out how much the patient understands of what he hears and why he cannot understand some of the language presented. He is asked to point to objects when they are named, then to pictures and to single words. Reduction of vocabulary comprehension may be noted if the patient can respond to words of a higher frequency of usage (hand, eye, nose) but fails to respond to words that are used less in everyday speech (elbow, eyebrow, forehead).

The patient is also asked to follow directions of increasing complexity. If auditory verbal retention has been impaired, he may be able to follow a simple command (point to the door), but be unable to follow a command of two or more steps (point to the picture of the car, then the bell, then the cat).

He may also be asked to respond to a question with the correct answer. If he cannot say it himself, a multiple-choice type of questioning may be used in which he is asked to respond

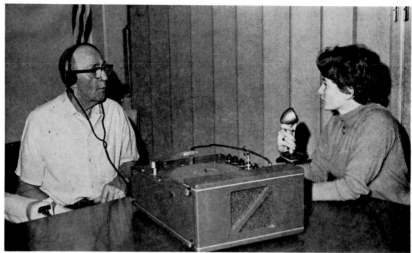

FIGURE 108. The auditory trainer provides amplification of sound and enhances concentration during a therapeutic session.

when he hears the correct answer to the question. Since this test is for auditory comprehension, no penalties are attached to the patient's inability to answer *verbally*.

The patient's reactions to normal conversation are also observed. When in the company of others he may react appropriately to jokes, comments and questions spoken to those around him, or he may show little or no recognition of this chatter as meaningful language.

Effective auditory stimulation must be used for both testing and treating patients. Auditory material presented to the patient must be short, meaningful and relevant (see Fig. 108).

Reading Comprehension

Visual acuity must be examined before the patient is requested to show his reading skills. Included in this examination is a determination of the patient's field of vision and whether there is any blurring, diplopia, or nystagmus which would interfere with his reading ability. If the patient wears glasses for reading, these are provided.

The patient is again asked to perform tasks which range from the simple to the complex. The patient's ability to recognize the correct printed word and more important, his ability to comprehend what he reads, are tested.

He is first requested to match geometric shapes. Although this sounds simple, the concept of matching like shapes or objects may prove impossible for the severely involved patient. He is then asked to match letters (a more complex series of geometric shapes). Any tendency to confuse letters of similar shapes should be noted. Such letter groups as E, L, F, T and B, P, R, and M, N, W, as well as lowercase groups of c, e, o and g, p, q, are especially confusing.

Next he is asked to match printed words with pictures of common objects. Any pictures presented should be realistic in context, proportion, and color. Cartoons and pictures in which figure-ground relationships may prove difficult should be avoided during initial testing.

The patient then is required to match the spoken word with the printed word. Again these should be words of high frequency usage which are familiar to the patient. Care should also be taken to test within the patient's educational level. If the patient has had sufficient schooling, words of higher grade level

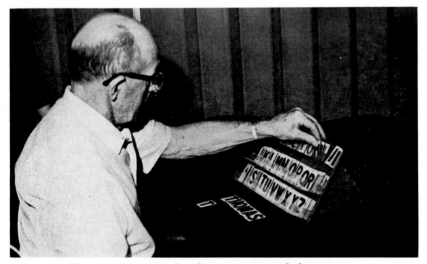

FIGURE 109. Visual aids may assist verbal responses.

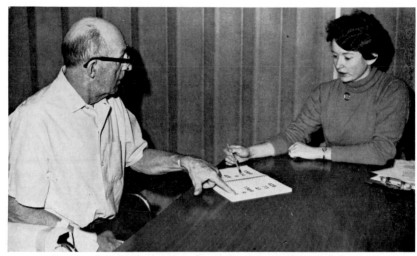

FIGURE 110.   Evaluating the ability to match visual forms.

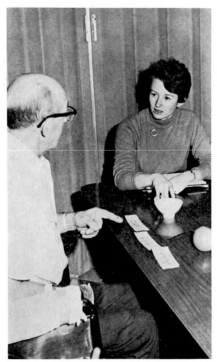

FIGURE 111.   Evaluating the ability to match objects to written words.

may be introduced. It should be noted whether the patient is able to read material commensurate with his educational and vocational background (see Figs. 109-111).

Sentences are then presented which may be read for content. Written questions may be used with a multiple-choice type of answer. The patient may be asked to read the question and find the correct answer. True-false statements may be presented which can be answered by yes or no.

Paragraphs chosen for increasing length and difficulty may be used. It is noted whether verbal retention remains constant or decreases as materials are made longer. A distinction should be made between the patient who reads slowly because he has difficulty recognizing the words and the one who must read the material over and over because he forgets what he has read (reduction of verbal retention span).

Testing the Speech Mechanism

The functions of speech are overlaid on body mechanisms which are primarily used for other purposes. The patient who has difficulty breathing, swallowing, and chewing will most likely also have a speech problem. If gross control of the muscles is affected, the finer movements needed for intelligible speech will also be impaired.

Paralysis or paresis of the pharyngeal musculature may often be determined by asking the patient if he has any difficulty eating and by confirming this by nurses' observations at mealtimes. This problem may or may not persist.

Some hemiplegic patients have a facial "droop" on the affected side. This area should be tested for movement patterns and for any sensory deficits. In more severe cases the larynx and the muscles of respiration may be involved.

The examiner may ask the patient to imitate movements of the tongue and jaw. The patient copies the motions for protruding and retracting the tongue, moving it laterally as well as from place to place inside the mouth on request. Rate of movement as well as accuracy of placement must be noted. The tongue that is weak will usually deviate toward the affected side since the stronger portion of the hypoglossus muscle continues to be innervated and overrides the movement of the weaker side of the tongue.

Rapid movements of the jaw such as those used in opening and closing the mouth quickly are checked. Any irregularity of movement should be investigated.

The patient is asked to repeat single words, phrases, and sentences. Any consistent articulation errors are noted. An introduction to self-corrective procedures may be attempted at this time by presenting the patient with correct auditory, visual, and tactile clues for the faulty sounds.

Voice problems may also exist. The patient's voice may be weak, breathy, or hoarse. He may have a monotonous pitch which he may not be able to raise or lower easily. His voice may taper off so that sentences are begun loudly but are barely audible several words later.

Dentures should be provided for those patients who wear them. Poor speech habits can be abetted by the absence of the customary dentures.

Evaluating the Use of Language

A unit of speech is one which is meaningful. Words uttered singly or in sequence are not a unit unless they are meaningful. Some patients with aphasia are able to produce automatic speech such as counting numbers or swearing but may be unable to speak the same words meaningfully. For example, a patient may be able to count from one to ten clearly but may be unable to tell the examiner how many fingers he has. Speech may be evoked from even extreme cases of aphasia, but it is not always meaningful.

The examiner may hear the patient say meaningful words and may be misled by these utterances into believing that the patient knows what he is saying. One patient for instance repeated the word "wonderful" for all speaking situations. If the examiner said "How are you?" her answer was relevant, but as future questioning was undertaken, it became obvious that the word was not meaningful *in context*.

The patient's language abilities are the major indicators of the type of degree of his aphasia. He may be able to use only single words, may respond yes and no appropriately, or may be able to use phrases or sentences.

A common problem is the "agrammatic" patient whose language consists of frequently- used nouns and simplified verb forms. He uses a limited number of structural patterns in a constricted vocabulary so that the resulting language often sounds "telegraphic" in that the connecting and modifying words are often omitted.

It is necessary to know how much language is available to the patient, how he uses this language to function in his environment, and how well he can organize his thoughts into words.

Upon greeting the patient, one notices whether he responds or attempts to respond. By asking questions which may be answered by one word, one can tell whether the patient is able to respond spontaneously or whether, as in many cases, he can recognize the correct answer but cannot recall the word without some prompting.

He may be asked to name common objects or parts of the body. The patient's errors may increase as the required words decrease in general frequency of usage. For example he may be able to name *eye* or *mouth*, but unable to name *eyebrow* or *lips*.

Asking the patient to describe the room may be helpful in determining his language abilities. Some patients tend to perseverate, that is, name one or more items over and over, rather than produce a catalog of the things they see. One patient became intrigued by the soundproofing panels on the ceiling to such an extent that he mentioned it six times and could not describe anything else in the room even when asked to look for other things. It is also important to note whether the patient is able to use modifying words (colors, numbers, qualities) or whether he relies on nouns. Does he use phrases or sentences?

The use of more complex language is tested by seeing whether he can define words he is familiar with or explain how two things are alike or different.

One can also ask the patient to give biographical information or to tell about his job and its various duties.

Evaluating the Patient's Ability to Write

Visuomotor disturbances as well as the hemiplegic's need to write with the nonpreferred hand may present additional problems to the aphasic patient when he is required to write. His writing may also show a reduction of language similar to that for oral tasks.

In offering the patient a pencil, one may see him attempt to use it with his preferred or his nonpreferred hand. He may have difficulty holding or guiding the pencil and may even write on the table next to the paper. In copying forms and letters, the patient with writing deficits may find it necessary to trace the pattern several times before he can produce it himself. Reversals of letters, confusion of similar letters, or distortion may also occur. He may indicate that he does not know how to start a letter or in which direction to proceed.

The patient often is able to write his name since this is a relatively automatic task. Asking him to write numbers or letters serially and then in random order may expose a reduction of his ability to attach a name to each symbol.

The patient's levels of written and oral spelling may be compared. He may show special difficulty with silent letters or double letters.

Further testing may consist of asking the patient to write sentences to dictation, then spontaneously to write paragraphs describing a picture. His educational level can then be compared with these efforts.

Other Language Activities

Many activities of daily living require the use of language skills. Those involving numbers are especially prevalent, such as telling time, dialing the telephone, using money, and cooking. Other activities include setting the dials for the oven, thermostat, or washing machine; selecting the correct floor in the elevator; writing checks, making bank deposits; or finding clothes of the correct size.

Many patients are able to sing although they may have no spontaneous speech. Group singing and conversation often help the patient to feel less alienated from others. Card games such as bridge or poker are still enjoyable to the patient who may have to point to his bid on a written list.

Prognostic Indicators

If patients are being considered for a rehabilitation program, attention should be given to their probable degree of success in such a program.

Anderson (1946) states the success of retraining a patient in speech therapy seems proportional to (1) the active cooperation of the patient, (2) his former training, (3) his morale, and (4) resolution of economic, personal, and social problems.

A good prognosis is indicated by a younger patient who has or had an outgoing personality, whose disturbance is associated with traumatic causes, who has modest aspiration levels, and whose training program was started early. A less hopeful prognosis is indicated by an older patient whose training is delayed, who has persistent euphoria, who has rigid or psychopathic tendencies, or who develops a great dependency on the clinician according to Eisenson (1949).

The premorbid personality may largely determine the maintenance of aphasia. Among chronic aphasics, Eisenson (1947) found a preponderance of higher ego-orientation, a higher proportion of excessively withdrawn individuals, or better adjustment to hospital than home situations, and a lower proportion of patients who felt loved or wanted at home.

Wepman (1958) states that the ability to recognize and self-correct errors is defective to some degree in almost every aphasic patient. He describes a continuum which ranges from those patients who cannot recognize their own errors and cannot correct them when they are pointed out to those patients who can and do recognize their errors and who correct them spontaneously. The speed with which the patient passes through the various stages of self-correction is seen as a prognostic indicator of his eventual level of recovery.

In an analysis of 122 aphasic patients whose ages ranged from sixteen to seventy-three years with a mean age of 52.7, Boone (1965) found age and etiology to have only random prognostic value. Individual screening tests were administered to patients at the beginning of treatment to predict how well a patient would speak at the end of language training. Two useful screening devices were found: (1) A pure-tone audiometric evaluation separated patients with gross intellectual deficits who could not follow audiometric procedures from true aphasic patients who gave reliable threshold responses. (2) Asking the patient to blow out a match revealed that those who were unable to do so had the poorest speech recoveries. Asking a patient to write his name proved unsuccessful as a screening device.

SPEECH THERAPY FOR THE APHASIC PATIENT

Preventing Frustration and Poor Speech Habits

During World War II, many brain-injured servicemen were sent to hospitals in hope that their language problems could be corrected as quickly as possible so that they could return to combat. Intensive therapy of three to seven hours a day with frequent rest periods and changes in the type of language stimulation were utilized benefically. It was generally found to be advantageous to start language therapy as soon after the injury as possible. Unfortunately, today many patients are less apt to receive prompt, intensive treatment with the result that they become accustomed to the feeling that speech is difficult to initiate, that their speech efforts are often ignored, and that they are not really expected to attempt communication.

In an autobiographical description of aphasia (Hall, 1961), a patient describes the initial events occurring around him as being "the way things were supposed to be," although speech had no meaning or function for him. He then began to understand the speech of others but could not make himself understood. This feeling of incompetence led to feelings of anger which could not be expressed.

The patient must adjust to different internal and external environmental conditions. In addition, many patients, especially in the early stages of their illness, feel that they have become insane or mentally incompetent. The anxiety created by this situation may become intolerable if it is not fully interpreted to the patient and to his family.

The patient must feel a need to communicate. All personnel

who come in contact with him must be urged to continue speech stimulation even if he seems unable to respond. The patient's slightest efforts at communication are commendable since he must feel that he can make himself understood by gesture, facial expression, or verbal response.

It is advisable that therapy be started as soon as possible after the acute phase of illness. Frustration and a sense of helplessness can be prevented if motivation for improvement is encouraged. A period of spontaneous recovery of speech, which is generally estimated to exist for three to six months, facilitates the early retraining of the aphasic patient.

The length of retraining required for maximum recovery of language functions is often one year or more. Since most patients are seen in a rehabilitation program for about three months, it may often be necessary to recommend further speech therapy on an outpatient basis, or it may be possible to set up a program which the family can carry out.

Therapy

Wepman (1953) presented a conceptual structure for aphasia therapy in which the primary function was a process by which the therapist provided stimulation in the area of a patient's greatest need, at a time when his nervous system was capable of integrating this material leading to language performance.

The best therapy uses the patient's abilities as a basis for training in those skills which he needs most for his immediate social demands. It consists of material with which he is familiar or which he must learn in order to perform easily in a hospital situation. A vocabulary of hospital words ("johnny," urinal, PT, OT, etc.) must be added to the existing list of items which he comprehends and possibly can say.

Clinical techniques will necessarily vary according to each patient's needs. Any technique may be useful but should be used with good judgment and for explicit purposes. Any technique, likewise, can be harmful or at least ineffectual if used indiscriminately.

Schuell, Jenkins and Jiménez-Pabón (1964) presented seven rules for increasing clinical effectiveness:

1. Talk simply and directly to the patient, eliminating extraneous noise that has no communicative value.
2. Control stimulation to elicit maximal response.
3. Control amount of material used and make it meaningful.
4. Use the principle of repeated stimulations to facilitate discrimination and recall.
5. Work to elicit a maximal number of responses. The patient should be responding continuously throughout the clinical period.
6. In general, restimulate rather than explain or correct.
7. Evaluate the effectiveness of each procedure with each patient.

The usual hospital clinic cannot provide enough speech and language training. Boone (1964) suggests the use of well-trained volunteers to aid in treating inpatients by providing more practice opportunities and by assuming the functions normally provided by the family in other settings. Aphasic patients can be helped by volunteers with language drills and with regular social conversational experiences. The volunteer's role is as an adjunct to the professional staff. The volunteers must adhere closely to the procedures outlined by the therapist.

Improving Auditory Comprehension

Auditory comprehension of spoken language is decreased in most or possibly all aphasic patients. The importance of auditory stimulation in therapy must therefore be emphasized.

Schuell (1953) based her therapy methods on auditory stimulation and found that patients improved in their abilities to talk, read, and write, in addition to their ability to understand. The patients progressed faster than previous patients had done when these tasks were treated as separate problems, and they seemed to have fewer difficulties in all areas.

Schuell's therapy techniques include the following:

1. Following directions.
2. Identifying objects in pictures.
3. Using overlearned language (automaticisms).
4. Repeating words.
5. Sentence completion.
6. Oral opposites.
7. Answering specific questions.
8. Naming pictures.
9. Identifying letters, words and sentences.
10. Reading in unison.

11. Listening to grasp the main idea.
12. Reading words and phrases.
13. Writing letters of the alphabet to dictation.
14. Spelling aloud.
15. Writing words to dictation.
16. Writing phrases and sentences to dictation.

All these tasks are increased in length and complexity as therapy progresses.

Taylor (1964) has found that exposure to language training improves the patient's auditory comprehension even if other modalities are not improved. The best improvement occurs when frequent, short periods of teaching are used, when the stimuli are exaggerated, and when each language task is broken down into its smallest linguistic units.

In a recent application of programmed instruction to speech therapy for aphasic patients, Taylor and Sands (1965) based their methodology on a stimulus-response theory in which patterned responses are conditioned to specified stimuli until these responses become automatic. Results of a preliminary study suggest that programmed instruction may be effective for teaching severely impaired brain-damaged subjects, including those with marked impairment of auditory comprehension and an absence of meaningful oral output.

Backus and Dunn (1947) found that auditory stimulation using "real speech" responses rather than drills speeded the transfer of normal speech production. The unit of speech used was the "phrase-response-in-a-situation."

Effective auditory stimulation consists of meaningful and relevant material. The length of each auditory unit must be carefully controlled. The patient should be actively involved in the therapeutic process and should be required to make a specific response to each language unit presented.

The Language Master (presently produced by Bell and Howell Company) is a useful visual and auditory aid. A portable device, it is activated by the insertion of a card on which is mounted a strip of sound tape. As the card makes contact, a voice pronounces words printed on the card while the patient sees the picture of an object and reads the printed word. Patients can be trained to operate the machine independently. They may

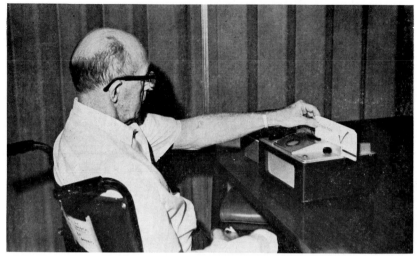

FIGURE 112.   Patient using the Language Master.

find it necessary at first to say the words with or after the taped voice and then may progress to reading the words orally before putting the card in the machine to verify their pronounciation (see Fig. 112).

The library of cards for the Language Master consists of six series, each with several sets of two hundred cards: The Vocabulary Builder Series, Word-Picture Series, Language Stimulation Series, English Development Series, Basic English Phonetics, and the Phonics Series.

Reading Skills

Reading skills in brain-damaged patients are often far below a level commensurate with their education and previous ability. Those who have visual field defects must be trained to read across the entire page; if this is not done, comprehension is severely affected by the words which are omitted.

Preliminary skills of matching are often utilized. Forms, letters, and words may be matched. It is often helpful to use picture cards on which appears a printed word. The patient begins by matching the picture and then becomes more aware of the printed word. A useful book is the *Puzzees Educational*

Aid Book One (1964), which includes push-out forms for matching colors, shapes, sizes, pictures, and forms.

The printed word may be matched with a picture of the object. The Taylor and Marks *Aphasia Rehabilitation Manual and Therapy Kit* (1959) consists of one hundred pictures of common objects and one hundred words on flashcards. These can be used in a variety of ways to facilitate reading and naming skills.

The spoken word may then be matched to the printed word. This task is more difficult because the stimulus must be retained by the patient; the stimulus, the spoken word, is not present in concrete form.

Look-alike words often cause difficulty. Longerich's *Manual for the Aphasic Patient* (1958) provides pages which have a picture and four similarly spelled responses, e.g., bid, bud, bed, bad.

As the patient increased his reading skills, a carefully controlled reading series such as the *Readers Digest Reading Skill Builder Series* is helpful. This series presents interesting, graded material with tests after many selections.

A weekly newspaper in two degrees of difficulty, *News For You,* provides current events in understandable versions.

Other materials can be devised and adapted by the therapist from magazines or books. Any material which is meaningful and relevant to the patient can be adapted to his present level of reading. This does not mean that difficult words cannot be presented. On the contrary, persons previously trained in any profession or trade can often respond to difficult passages pertaining to their field of work.

Speech Mechanisms

Some patients are unable to produce any sounds upon request but phonate normally when they cough, cry, or laugh. The patient can be instructed by placing his hand on the therapist's larynx to feel it vibrate and then on his own larynx. The first phonation, no matter how feeble should be praised. Asking the patient to produce open vowels or to hum are the next steps.

Manipulation of the tongue for simple placement, pressure,

and agility exercises are beneficial. Some patients seem to have little idea how to move their tongues or where their tongues are. Mirror work for protrusion and lateralization of the tongue are helpful.

Speech movements can often be elicited by asking the patient to produce automatic series, such as counting or saying the days of the week. Nonsense syllables are usually of little value since they have no significance to the patient. Simple combinations of sounds that *are* words can be used, such as me, my, arm, pop, pie, pea, bee, by, bow, ear, eye.

For patients who have difficulty pronouncing certain speech sounds simple instruction in the placement of the speech articulators is used. Tactile stimulation, visual and auditory clues help the patient correct his errors.

Writing

Hemiplegic patients often must learn to write with their nonpreferred hand. Gross control of arm and hand muscles is taught by the occupational therapist before the finer movements necessary for writing can be undertaken.

The patient is asked to copy forms and letters and to write his name (a relatively automatic task). Look-alike letters will often cause difficulty at first. The patient is asked to write letters and numbers to dictation. Spelling skills are also taught.

Taylor and Sands (1965) found that severely brain-damaged patients were often able to write long before they were able to respond orally. They express the hypothesis that perhaps writing is a paralanguage skill.

Oral Language Skills

Taylor (1964a) notes that the order in which the various parts of speech are recovered appears to respect the order of loss. From the first to be relearned to the last they are nouns, verbs, adverbs, adjectives, prepositions, pronouns, conjunctions, and articles.

Language tasks may first concentrate on naming simple nouns and verbs. Several sets of picture cards are available which have both the picture and the printed word. The patient listens to the word until he feels that he is able to say it. If his pronounciation approximates the correct sounds, it is accepted without correction. He is then asked to name the pictures without auditory clues if possible. When this is accomplished, questions involving a choice of previously learned words are employed such as "What do you wear on your head? What do you sleep in?" These questions lead to having the patient complete a phrase such as, you sleep in a *bed;* a cup of *coffee;* green *grass;* light a *match;* smoke a *cigarette;* look out a *window.* At this point the Language Master may be employed to provide additional stimulation.

Asking the patient to define words which he should know will give indications of his ability to recall synonyms and to associate ideas. He may provide chance association, or he may use phrases and sentences which accurately define the word.

The patient's ability to use sentences varies from a two-word form, "I eat, boy runs," etc., to an ability to use modifying words, articles, and prepositions correctly.

More advanced tasks include asking the patient to explain similarities between two objects, to describe pictures, and to retell paragraphs which he follows while the therapist reads.

Unfortunately all patients with language disturbances do not recover sufficient ability to communicate. The speech therapist judges progress and prognosis carefully in order to enlighten the rest of the team. Constant advice is available to team members which frequently helps advance their programs with the patient as well. The speech therapist also devotes time to the patient's family as discharge approaches to assist the transition from hospital to home life.

REFERENCES

AGRANOWITZ, ALEEN, AND McKEOWN, MILFRED R.: *Aphasia Handbook.* Springfield, Thomas, 1964.

ANDERSON, JEANETT O.: *Is* is not the verb for aphasia. *J Speech Dis,* 11:135, 1946.

ANDERSON, JEANETTE O.: The speech examination of aphasic patients. *J Speech Dis,* 7:361, 1942.

BACKUS, OLLIE L.: The rehabilitation of aphasic veterans. *J Speech Dis,* 10:149, 1945.

BACKUS, OLLIE L., AND DUNN, HARRIET: Use of conversational patterns to promote speed and retention of learning. *J Speech Dis, 12*:135, 1947.

BERRY, MILDRED F., AND EISENSON, JON: *Speech Disorders.* New York, Appleton, 1956.

BIORN-HANSEN, VERA: Social and emotional aspects of aphasia. *J Speech Hearing Dis, 22*:53, 1957.

BOONE, DANIEL R.: Prognostic Determinants in Aphasia. Talk given at Amer. Speech Hearing Assoc. Convention, Nov. 1, 1965. (41st Annual Convention, Chicago.)

BOONE, DANIEL R.: The use of volunteers in the speech pathology-audiology clinic in the medical setting. *ASHA, 6*:284, 1964.

BROWN, JOE R., AND SCHUELL, HILDRED: A preliminary report of a diagnostic test for aphasia. *J Speech Hearing Dis, 15*:21, 1950.

EISENSON, JON: Aphasics: Observations and tentative conclusions. *J Speech Dis, 12*:290, 1947.

EISENSON, JON: Prognostic factors related to language rehabilitation in aphasic patients. *J Speech Hearing Dis, 14*:262, 1949.

GESCHWIND, NORMAN: The test of time. VIII. Aphasia. *Boston Med Quart, 16*:129, 1965.

GODA, SIDNEY: Spontaneous speech, a primary source of therapy material. *J Speech Hearing Dis, 27*:190, 1962.

GOLDSTEIN, KURT: *After Effects of Brain Injuries in War.* New York, Grune, 1942.

GOLDSTEIN, KURT: *Language and Language Disturbances.* New York, Grune, 1948.

HALL, ALONZO: Return from silence—A personal experience. *J Speech Hearing Dis, 26*:174, 1961.

HALPER, ANITA: Speech therapy and stroke victims. *RIC Report,* Chicago, no date.

HALSTEAD, W. C., AND WEPMAN, J. M.: *The Halstead-Wepman Screening Test for Aphasia.* Chicago, U. of Chicago Clinics, 1949.

HUBER, MARY: Linguistic problems of brain-injured servicemen. *J Speech Dis, 11*:143, 1946.

JOHNSON, WENDELL; DARLEY, FREDRIC L., AND SPRIESTERSBACH, D. C.: *Diagnostic Methods in Speech Pathology.* New York, Harper, 1963, pp. 185-187.

LONGERICH, MARY C.: *Manual for the Aphasia Patient.* New York, Macmillan, 1958.

LONGERICH, MARY C., AND BORDEAUX, JEAN: *Aphasia Therapeutics.* New York, Macmillan, 1954.

MILLER, MAURICE H.: Audiologic evaluation of aphasic patients. *J Speech Hearing Dis, 25*:333, 1960.

News For You. Syracuse, N. Y., Laubach Literacy, Inc., 1966.

PETERSON, JEAN C., AND OLSEN, ANN P.: *Language Problems After a Stroke.* Minneapolis, Sister Kenny Foundation, 1964.

Puzzees Educational Aid Book One, William A. Adams, Ed. Detroit, Perception Aid, 1964.

Reader's Digest Reading Skill Builder Series. Pleasantville, N. Y., Reader's Digest Services, 1958.

RUSSELL, W. R., AND ESPIR, M. L. E.: *Traumatic Aphasia.* London, Oxford, 1961.

SCHUELL, HILDRED: Auditory impairment in aphasia: Significance and retraining techniques. *J Speech Hearing Dis, 18*:14, 1953.

SCHUELL, HILDRED: *The Minnesota Test for Differential Diagnosis of Aphasia.* Minneapolis, U. of Minn., 1965.

SCHUELL, HILDRED: A re-evaluation of the short examination for aphasia. *J Speech Hearing Dis, 31*:137, 1966.

SCHUELL, HILDRED; CARROLL, VIRGINIA, AND STREET, BARBARA S.: Clinical treatment of aphasia. *J Speech Hearing Dis, 20*:43, 1955.

SCHUELL, HILDRED; JENKINS, JAMES J., AND JIMÉNEZ-PABÓN, EDWARD: *Aphasia in Adults: Diagnosis, Prognosis, and Treatment.* New York, Harper, 1964.

SHEEHAN, VIVIAN M.: Techniques in the management of aphasics. *J Speech Hearing Dis, 13*:241, 1948.

SIES, LUTHER, AND BUTLER, RICHARD: A personal account of dysphasia. *J Speech Hearing Dis, 28*:261, 1963.

SIMON, CLARENCE T.: Comments on testing aphasics in the speech clinic. *J Speech Dis, 11*:139, 1946.

TAYLOR, MARTHA L.: Linguistic considerations of the verbal behavior of the brain damaged adult. *Linguistic Reporter, 6*:1, 1964(a).

TAYLOR, MARTHA L.: A Measurement of Functional Communication in Aphasia. Paper presented to Amer. Academy of Phys. Med. and Rehab., Boston, Aug. 24, 1964(b).

TAYLOR, MARTHA L., AND MARKS, MORTON: *Aphasia Rehabilitation Manual and Therapy Kit.* New York, McGraw, 1959.

TAYLOR, MARTHA L., AND SANDS, ELAINE: Application of Programmed Instruction Techniques to the Language Rehabilitation of Severely Impaired Aphasic Adults. Paper presented at the 41st annual convention of the Amer. Speech and Hearing Assoc., Chicago, October 31, 1965.

TRAVIS, LEE E. (ED).: *Handbook of Speech Pathology,* New York, Appleton, 1957.

TYLER, H. RICHARD: Modern concepts of the pathenogenesis, diagnosis and treatment of cerebrovascular accidents. *Med Clin N Amer, 44*:1215, 1960.

WEPMAN, JOSEPH: A conceptual model for the processes involved in recovery from aphasia. *J Speech Hearing Dis, 18*:4, 1953.

WEPMAN, JOSEPH: The language disorders. In *Psychological Practices with the physically Disabled,* James Garrett and Edna Levine, Eds. New York, Columbia, 1962, pp. 197-230.

WEPMAN, JOSEPH: The organization of therapy for aphasia: I. The in-patient treatment center. *J Speech Dis, 12*:405, 1947.

WEPMAN, JOSEPH: *Recovery from Aphasia.* New York, Ronald, 1951.

WEPMAN, JOSEPH: The relationship between self-correction and recovery from aphasia. *J Speech Hearing Dis, 23*:302, 1958.

WEPMAN, JOSEPH, AND JONES, LYLE V.: *Studies in Aphasia: An Approach to Testing: The Language Modalities Test for Aphasia,* Chicago, Education Industry Service, 1961.

WEPMAN, JOSEPH, AND MORENCY, ANNE: Filmstrips as an adjunct to language therapy for aphasia. *J Speech Hearing Dis, 28*:191, 1963.

Chapter XI

ROLE OF THE SOCIAL WORKER

T ODAY'S CHALLENGE TO the social worker in the health field appears to be, in conjunction with the medical team, the preservation of the health of the citizen, singly and collectively. Comprehensive health care requires not only the services of the physician and his team of health workers, but also the resources of the community to achieve positive health and to prevent or treat illness and disability. Medical social workers are committed to the objective of positive health and are therefore expected to cooperate with and participate in Out Patient, Home Care, and other community health programs when they are set up by public or private medical institutions or agencies. Their preventive approach to patients in seeking early diagnosis, treatment, and the lessening of disability, makes rehabilitation a most natural area for their constant effort and achievement.

The function of the social worker as a team member in a rehabilitation center differs little from his function in a social agency. The focus of his involvement is the client who may be a patient on the ward or in the clinic. He requires the same knowledge of human growth and behavior from the physical, psychological, emotional, and social points of view and the same knowledge of motivations which influence patterns of behavior and use of medical care. He is knowledgeable concerning the effect of grief reactions resulting from loss of relatives, friends, limbs, or employment; and about the medical care community, as well as the cultural influences in the patient's background. Frequent focusing on the emotional components of various disabilities, however, may increase her skill in treating problems of physical rehabilitation.

The clinical or medical social worker in a rehabilitation center has an excellent opportunity to practice preventive casework as well as to intervene in crisis situations. The stroke patient and members of his family often benefit by interviews with the social worker as soon as admission procedures are completed. Review of his application, interagency referral form, or even summaries by letter or telephone may alert the social worker to a serious disability or social dysfunctioning. He may then initiate contact with the patient or any appropriate collateral person or agency to begin his study of the social situation. He need not wait for the physician or other member of the health team to refer a patient to him for service after a problem has been presented by the patient, his family, or someone in the community.

The trained social worker employs three treatment methods in his effort to help the stroke patient in a rehabilitation setting. The first of these, social casework, is a method of study, diagnosis, and treatment of problems which is based on understanding of human behavior. This is used by trained medical social workers in hospitals and rehabilitation centers. It is a helping process with a goal of enabling the patient to deal with his psychosocial problems in such a way as to relieve stress and to improve social functioning. The social worker seeks to understand the patient's viewpoint. This requires the development of a professional relationship between them which permits the patient to express his feelings, and at a tempo geared to his readiness. The areas included under casework are those in which the problem and treatment call for a one-to-one relationship between the social worker and the individual with the problem.

Social work with groups is a second method used in helping stroke patients. Social workers have treated groups in many settings, and medical social workers have worked with patients and their families in groups for many years. They are now endeavoring to broaden the scope of their efforts with groups of patients to benefit the hospital and the community as well. Although some exploring of group approaches is permissable, the social worker treating a group of stroke patients has the same responsibility as the caseworker to relate her activity to comprehensive health goals. In a 65-bed rehabilitation center, however, where the average length of stay is less than four months, casework remains the dominant method.

Another widely accepted method of social work in the health field is community organization. Social workers in all health agencies are in strategic positions to identify, evaluate, and document social problems affecting health. They can then endeavor to discover ways of preventing them, establish new services, and strengthen those already in existence. When a stroke patient has received maximum benefit from the rehabilitation program and is ready to return to the community, the need for such services may arise. Occasionally a public health or visiting nurse's service may be essential. More frequently it is a home health aide or attendant who is needed. Suitable recreation also should be available to those disabled by a stroke. When local facilities, services, and needs can be evaluated, the appropriate community resources may be supplemented through local community service agencies.

The distinctive characteristic of social casework in a medical or health setting is its collaboration with medical and related professional personnel. The social worker participates in the teamwork process which involves the physician-in-charge, the rehabilitation nurse, the physical therapist, the occupational therapist, and the speech therapist, as well as the dentist, the psychiatrist, the podiatrist, and any other treating the patient. It is important for him to know and appreciate the subculture of medicine, the authority of the physician, and the complexities of the doctor-patient realtionship. Respect for and acceptance of the other team members plus the appropriate timing of activity in relation to their readiness are essential. Also important for effective teamwork are the social worker's own self-awareness and disciplined professional relationships.

Consultation is considered to be an important indirect service function of the social worker in medical care facilities. In a rehabilitation setting particularly, it is a process predicated upon mature professional competence and acceptance of other disciplines in their own roles. Interprofessional consultation can be vital in treating and planning with a stroke patient. It is essential that the social worker in a consultant role be willing and able to leave the responsibility for seeking and using consultation to the consultee. The aim of the social worker as a consultant is always that of furthering the ability of the consultee to understand and to deal with a problem presented by a patient.

When the stroke patient is admitted to the rehabilitation ward the nurse who takes responsibility for assigning him to a room and giving him whatever immediate care may be required often gives the social worker his first leads about the patient as a person. The nurse also has the first contact with a person or persons who may accompany the patient to the rehabilitation center. Usually after explaining some of the routine requirements including appropriate clothing for therapy sessions, she will refer this person to the social worker for further orientation and the beginning of a social study of the patient. Often the social worker is enabled at this early stage to get a picture of the family's or society's attitude toward the patient's disability and learn about the pressures—social, economic and psychological—which are bearing down on the new patient.

Early contact with the closest relative or friend of the patient can be vital because what has happened to the patient has undoubtedly affected the total family group. They too may have suffered severe trauma and need help in readjusting. An admission interview may be the first step in an effort to restore family equilibrium and prepare them to accept the patient again as a functioning part of the family or community. They may need immediate help with their anxiety and assurance that the staff is interested in them as well as the patient. This may be the time to prevent any feeling that the patient has become entirely the hospital's responsibility.

The sooner the social worker's study of the stroke patient can start after his admission to the rehabilitation center, the better. It is usually his first experience in such a setting and it can be a very devastating one. If patients come from a local area and have heard that the hospital is primarily for chronic or terminal care, this requires interpretation. Fear is a usual reaction to a major stroke, and this may be intensified by anxiety about the possibility of being rejected by one's family and left to die in the hospital. Thus a crisis situation often exists at time of admission indicating a need for the social worker's intervention as early as possible even though the acute phase of the stroke may have passed. This is the time for the social worker to offer help and support in order to prevent reactions, attitudes, and plans which, once established, will hamper the patient's progress toward the therapeutic goals.

Study of the stroke patient's current medical-social situation is necessary before casework treatment can be offered to the patient or his family. From the application for admission the social worker can obtain the previous physician's diagnosis and description of the disability. At the staff evaluation conference when the patient is presented to the physician-in-charge of the rehabilitation center, the social worker can observe his responses or lack of them. The patient may then need help to objectively examine himself and the situation in which he finds himself. If he is nonverbal, the social study may be a long slow process and one that can be accomplished only through collaboration with the speech therapist or other staff person on whom he may be more dependent for help.

An understanding of the patient's characteristics and capacities as a person is very important to the social worker. He notes the patient's reactions, feelings, beliefs, and attitudes, as evidenced in his recent life situation and as seen in his current behavior as a stroke patient. Significant factors in this assessment relate to how he sees himself, what value he places on physical functioning, his goals and ambitions, and his ability to face life's problems realistically. This appraisal may reveal the seriousness of the stroke to the particular patient, and his particular strengths which may affect his ability and motivation to invest in efforts toward overcoming his handicap.

The social worker's evaluation of the patient's achievements and limitations in areas of economic matters, housing arrangements, education, health, employment, recreation and personal-social relationships should be shared with the therapeutic team early in the program. He should be ready to share with all the team members his assessment of the environmental and the personal-social problems resulting from the patient's disability. He must also attempt to assess the patient's strengths in coping with problems, his attitude toward his disability, the level of his motivation, and his goals in rehabilitation. His approach should include the family's attitudes and ability to help the patient achieve his goals.

At admission or shortly thereafter, the social worker needs

to assess the mood of the patient as he may be facing a period of mourning if he does not begin to regain function in a paralyzed leg or arm. In addition, many patients 60 years of age or over have lost a husband, wife, or parent in recent years and the grief over loss of function is superimposed on the personal loss. Perhaps the most frustrating situation of all is that of the wage earner who loses his speech in addition to the use of his arm or leg and sees himself chiefly as a burden to his family. He and his family may have seen a rehabilitation program as the means to get him back to independent functioning and even to employment. When this does not develop, the therapeutic team may have to deal with anxiety, guilt, inferiority, frustration, and depression.

The more positive relationships the patient has, the better is his prognosis for adjustment. The social worker therefore must not only study the patient as a person with a disability in order to offer casework treatment, but must provide the other staff members with pertinent psychosocial information so that the most effective rehabilitation program possible may be planned. He must determine his role with the patient's family and with the community. This may range from promoting awareness of psychosocial factors to enabling a family member to cope with the current problems and move ahead with planning, or to finding a community agency to provide service and assist in the maintenance of the patient's rehabilitation gains. Thus the social worker endeavors to fulfill a liaison role with the therapeutic team, with the patient's family, and with the community.

The social worker's first aim in treatment of the stroke patient is to lessen the worry and anxiety besetting him. He can be the sounding board of reality against which the patient and his family can test their fears, their feelings, or responsibility for his plight, and their ideas about what needs to be done to help the patient receive maximum benefit from treatment. He takes time in interviews to listen to the details of present concerns, the telling of which relieves pent-up feelings. He sifts possible courses of action regarding present and acute needs. He acts particularly to delay major changes in life plans until the full recovery potential of the patient can be known. Precipitous planning can have a disastrous effect on the patient and his future social recovery.

Casework treatment is aimed at the solution or alleviation of social problems and the achievement and maintenance of rehabilitation goals. It may take several forms such as assisting the patient to deal with his dependency, hostility, resistance, and concern with his disability; encouraging the patient to sustain hope and realize his essential value to others; aiding him to discover new interests and capacities, or helping the family to see him as a decreasingly dependent individual, with acknowledgment of his new abilities.

The social worker needs to delineate the characteristics of the stroke patient and his situation which indicate to what extent the principal procedures of casework can be of value in treatment. The treatment of a stroke patient may be an individualized blend of procedures, themes, and goals. Choice and emphasis by the social worker should follow definite principles and rest upon most careful evaluation of (1) the nature of his problem, (2) external and internal causative factors and their modifiability, (3) the patient's motivation, and (4) pertinent aspects of his personality. The evaluative process is an ongoing one, with the emphasis in treatment varying in harmony with the changing needs and capacities of the patient.

One of the social worker's goals with the stroke patient is that of helping him to gain self-acceptance as well as acceptance by his family or a key person. This goal is often a difficult one to attain and the degree of success differs from patient to patient as does the psychological makeup of each patient. Encouraging and strengthening attitudes on the part of the patient which lead to increased motivation and participation in planning his own program are objectives of the social worker in common with other team members. He appropriately gives continued interpretation of the methods and objectives of the rehabilitation program. He plans with the patient, and usually the family, the means to carry out staff recommendations. In order to function effectively, he must frequently coordinate the rehabilitation services prescribed for the patient.

The observations of the therapists in their continuous daily activities with the stroke patient are extremely important for the social worker to know as an additional means of understanding the patient and his needs. Prolonged and strong relationships with staff therapists can be used constructively by the social worker to enable the patient to focus on and attain suitable social goals. Patients do not ordinarily come to rehabilitation centers for social or psychological help, but for physical restoration, speech and hearing therapy, or possibly preparation for vocational training. Here they find a team of professional helping persons. Sometimes a helping person does not take into sufficient account the stroke patient's feelings, his readiness, his capacity, and his right to be actively involved in the helping process. When a patient is not adjusting satisfactorily to the rehabilitation program, the social worker's assistance may be enlisted to enable the patient to better utilize the offered services or to help the team to understand and better manage his resistances.

A social service case conference is often used to advantage by the staff to promote understanding of the patient by the team working directly with him. By limiting attendance at this conference to those who work directly with the patient in a treatment role, more confidential material can be shared which may be essential to the understanding and acceptance of a patient's behavior, or the planning proposed by the social worker. To make these conferences effective, the social worker must be capable of making sound judgments and taking responsibility for setting social goals in line with the patient's wishes and his capacities. In the long run, the social worker's essential contribution may be his steady work toward making knowledge and understanding of psychosocial factors more vital and more truly operative in the comprehensive care of the patient. It is only when the knowledge contributed by the social worker is used by the team in setting therapeutic goals and when it affects the day-to-day relationship of the team members with the patient that a truly comprehensive program is in operation.

Before undertaking group therapy it is important to know the dynamics of grouping as well as the dynamics of the individual patient. Weekly group sessions led by a social worker consist of five, or more women or men with stroke. The purpose of the group includes socialization, adjustment to the rehabilitation center, sharing of common and unique problems with ventilation of frustrations, and mutual support and encouragement in planning for the future. In spite of the fact that the group changes because of admission and discharge of patients from the rehabilitation center, an *esprit de corps* develops among the patients participating in it and they usually appreciate the extra opportunity for self-expression. Out of group sessions also it is found that changes for the better in overall hospital or ward policies and procedures occasionally develop.

Any service to seriously disabled patients requires the utmost conviction about the basic impulse to growth which the social work profession holds is inherent in human beings. The social worker treating the hemiplegic patient must not only hold that particular conviction, but must be able to convey it to the patient and to the team. He must strive for more precise identification of the level where the patient's motivation lies for that is where he must take hold in order to start to help the patient. He needs to analyze thoroughly and carefully the resources within the patient and outside the patient, in his family, community, or in the center itself which can be stimulated to enhance his functioning according to his capacities.

Another extremely important aspect of treatment is the use of casework techniques to enable the stroke patient and his family, in preparation for his discharge from the rehabilitation center, to make the best use of resources in the community. At this point the social worker needs to be an integrator of services to facilitate the patient's transition from being a patient to being a person again. When the patient has received what appears to be maximum benefit from the rehabilitation program, the social worker's activities are related to the patient's need for normal social living, or the closest approximation to this consistent with his physical status. Human beings need a well-rounded life for a feeling of well-being, so the social worker is challenged to think in terms of what social deficits there are in a particular stroke patient's life situation, and in what way his physical abilities can be supplemented to give him the fullest life possible.

Assessment of the possible consequences for the patient and

his family of a proposed course of action is essential in advance of the patient's discharge from the rehabilitation center to avoid failure of a discharge plan, especially the disruption of a home care plan because of poor family relationships. For instance, a social worker often has the responsibility to help a married son or daughter of a patient who has not attained independence in activities of daily living to decide whether he or she can with goodwill take the patient home and make his or her few remaining years as comfortable as possible. When this action would obviously impose too great a burden on the patient's family, the social worker must try to help the responsible son or daughter face the reality of the situation and take responsibility for making an alternate plan with or for the patient. Every effort must always be made to enable the patient to participate in the decision making and the planning.

When the extent of the patient's physical disability, the nature of his emotional attitude, or the socioeconomic situation, point to the need for his placement in a nursing home after a rehabilitation effort, the social worker may have an extremely difficult task to help the patient and his family accept such a plan. All the negative thoughts and feelings of a lifetime about nursing homes may have to be aired and worked through before the patient and family can begin to move toward acceptance of nursing home care. Uprooting the older patient from his own home and lifelong neighborhood may expose him to severe emotional shock. Therefore the choice of a nursing home where his needs and standards will best be met is quite crucial. Conscientious relatives may need support to overcome feelings of guilt about the decision to place the patient.

If the patient is not too brain-damaged, his participation in the planning and in selecting the appropriate nursing home can gradually lessen his resistance to the proposed change and may prevent his emotional deterioration. The social worker helps those concerned with the patient base their judgments of nursing homes on relevant factors rather than superficial ones. The nursing home staff may also be helped to recognize that a patient's anger may be a defense against his anxiety and that aggressive behavior often covers feelings of rejection; that the patient's excessive complaints and demands may be related to his fear of loss of control; and that his depression may be related to loss of close relationships or possessions. The social worker always looks for the causes of difficult behavior which may be easily modifiable when understood.

It is quite essential that the social worker on the team treating stroke patients be aware of community resources and well informed about all aspects of financial assistance programs. Many patients have to apply for disability assistance or medical assistance by the time an application is filed for their admission to a rehabilitation center. The physician and therapists therefore look to the social worker to coordinate their requests for authorization of aids to promote the patients' progress in ambulation and self-care activities. These include orthopedic shoes, braces, walkers, and quad canes; also grab bars, safety rails, and railings for installation in bathrooms and stairways at home. The social worker needs to be aware of the channels through which requests for such items are processed in order to contact the right persons at the right time to expedite provision of the required items; otherwise, patients may become depressed, discouraged, or even hostile if their hospital stay is prolonged by a delay.

Helping a patient overcome hostile or negative feelings about accepting assistance from public programs is a frequent function of the social worker. Since financial independence is often considered a measure of personal adequacy, a hemiplegic patient may be too sensitive and insecure to accept help. Self-concept includes both body image and the patient's conception of himself as a social being. By listening and creating a climate of respect and understanding, the social worker may enable patients or their families to move toward acceptance of the maximum assistance to which they are entitled.

By adequate communication with his colleagues in community social agencies, the social worker can prepare them for the patient's discharge from the rehabilitation center and increase their readiness to continue supportive help be it medical, social, emotional, or financial. Most vital may be the social worker's interpretation to an untrained public assistance worker who may be strategically placed for secondary prevention. The local social worker often wants and needs to know more about a stroke patient and what is necessary for maintenance of the gains from a rehabilitation program. The Visiting Nurse may profit considerably, if she has not known the patient prior to his stroke, by social information in addition to the physician's orders and the rehabilitation nurse's outline of care and recommendations.

As a younger stroke patient approaches physical readiness for vocational counseling and training, it is incumbent on the social worker to assist the team in assessment of his social and emotional readiness for work or training. Occasionally he finds that a patient who is determined to return to the same firm for which he formerly worked succeeds in doing so in spite of its apparent unsuitability at the time of discharge from the rehabilitation program. Union protection and sometimes longevity of employment will facilitate necessary adjustments, and the patient will be rehired and helped to adjust until the minimum retirement age is reached. Those younger and more severely disabled patients whom the social worker refers to the rehabilitation commission often need continued supportive help until they are actively involved in the vocational rehabilitation process whether it be training, sheltered workshop, or steady employment.

When a hemiplegic patient has been treated in physical therapy or occupational therapy long enough to determine that he is likely to have residual disability at the time of discharge from the rehabilitation program, the team is alerted and the social worker explores the possibility of a home visit by his therapists before his discharge. This service is necessarily restricted to patients who live in communities within easy distance of the hospital. The social worker may have already informed anxious relatives that such a service is available, but if not, he proposes it at this point to reassure the family that we wish to help them safeguard the comfort and safety of the patient at home and help him to maintain the gains made on our program. Occasionally the social worker may get a negative reaction to a proposed home visit when the patient, who also goes on the home visit, has related poorly to the staff, or if relatives feel that we are underestimating their ability to prepare for the patient's homecoming.

When the social worker has developed a strong relationship with a patient, he is in a strategic position not only to offer him continued emotional support but to give the understanding and support needed by a family facing the stress of supervision at home of a patient who cannot attain the goal of complete independence. If there is a problem around family interrelationships or if a homemaker or home aide is placed in the home, the social worker may plan to visit the home with a nurse or therapist or on his own. He may thereby get a clearer social picture of the patient's place in the family, the degree of family unity, the overt stresses and strains in the home environment, and the degree of flexibility of the environment for possible change. Usually it is not necessary for the social worker to make the home visit, but rather to help the patient and family carry out the staff recommendations resulting from the home visit. Frequently he keeps active in the situation following the patient's discharge until a followup visit is made a month or so later to determine whether an effective, realistic discharge paln has been made. It has been noted that the return to a familiar physical and social environment is particularly important to the hemiplegic patient.

Education of the patient and his family about community resources may commence upon his application or admission to the rehabilitation center as he may have been financially as well as physically independent before his stroke. Although the admission or credit office may refer the patient's family or responsible person to the welfare department if eligibility for a program of medical assistance is indicated, the social worker frequently has to handle the feelings aroused by such a referral. Anxiety about discharge from the rehabilitation program before the goal of independence is attained is often tied in with feelings of inferiority because of dependence on a public program. The rehabilitation social worker needs not only knowledge of the benefit to which patients and their families are entitled, but faith and confidence in the value of life itself in order to help patients with severe residuals of a stroke achieve a feeling of dignity, worth, and some self-determination.

The social worker's role of interpretation to the community of the needs of the stroke patient is a constant one. Since the patient's relatives are part of the community, the social worker aims to develop their confidence in the rehabilitation program and encourage their cooperation in discharge planning. The social worker usually proposes that relatives who are resistant to the discharge of a dependent patient meet the patient's therapists and learn what the patient is able to do for himself. The social worker can discuss with the family what help may be available for them in the community to help them provide adequate care and a satisfying social situation for the patient. When the patient does not have a family, the social worker naturally takes over more responsibility for planning with him.

Communities vary widely in their medical and social agency resources. Such areas as diet counseling, weight control, exercise, foot care, hygiene, and prevention of complications may require followup by the Visiting Nurse Association or Public Health Nurses. A Homemaker or Home Health Aide may be essential, and the availability of such service is very uneven. Continued social casework, physical, occupational, and speech therapy may be recommended, particularly speech, which may have responded the least to therapy while the patient remained at the center. Help with housing may be essential to the patient who has had to give up an apartment or house during a prolonged hospitalization. Recreational programs may also be a vital need. The social worker has the responsibility to bring omissions in community service to the attention of those involved in community planning as related to the interests of the hospital and rehabilitation center. He acknowledges that success in the social rehabilitation of a stroke patient is measured not by his willingness and ability to adapt himself to an unnecessarily restricted world, but by the extent to which his maximum inherent social capacities are realized.

It is evident from the nature of the responsibilities of a social worker on the team treating the stroke patient that he is also expected to serve on social action committees, to participate in local organizations promoting health and medical care, and to speak on panels describing his role on the therapeutic team of the rehabilitation center. He is expected to cooperate at all times with public and private health organizations operating broad programs of prevention, community services, professional education, and community research. He makes available social-aspect material to other health professions and shares knowledge with the various disciplines in his collaborative work on behalf of patients.

The experienced clinical social worker usually has teaching responsibilities with student groups in the rehabilitation setting. These may be primarily with nursing students and physical and occupational therapy students. At least one orientation session is given to each group of nursing students assigned to the rehabilitation ward, the major objective of which is to increase their understanding of the effects of disability and hospitalization on patients and their families. Orientation and teaching of therapy students is mostly by the conference method when various aspects of the stroke patient's problems may be discussed. These sessions may help the therapists understand and modify attitudes toward a troubled patient. The social worker must also be prepared to provide field instruction or summer experience for social work students and to supervise trained social workers who are new in a medical rehabilitation setting.

A rehabilitation center offers the social worker opportunities to observe stroke patients over an average of three to four months and to participate in multidisciplinary studies of the effects of treatment on these patients, their families, and the community. His share in research activity is focused on the social factors affecting the patient's disability, while independent social work research is interested in examining the social work process in order to increase knowledge about effective casework treatment of patients. It is the social worker's aim to improve his practice in order to increase his contribution to the patient's well-being. He ideally should be able to engage in research to validate his impression of the influences of social situations on motivation and the attainment of rehabilitation goals. Participation in research should assist the social worker in determining the services and methods which best meet human needs and thereby increase his effectiveness in working with the patient, the family, the community, and the therapeutic team.

REFERENCES

BARTLETT, HARRIETT M.: *Social Work Practice in the Health Field.* New York, Nat. Assn. of Social Workers, 1961, pp. 102, 120, 236.

BARTLETT, HARRIET M.: The widening scope of hospital social work. *Social Casework, 44*(1):10, 1963.

COCKERILL, ELEANOR E., AND GOSSETT, HELEN M.: Social services in stroke care. *J Rehabil, 29*(6):43, United States Department of Health, Education and Welfare.

FARRAR, MARCELLA; RYDER, MARGARET B., AND BLENKNER, MARGARET: Social work responsibility in nursing home care. *Social Casework, 45*(9):532, 1964.

FREY, LOUISE A. (Ed.): *Use of Groups in the Health Field.* Report of the Committee on the Utilization of Group Methods in the Health Field. New York, Nat. Assn. of Social Workers, 1966, p. 9.

HAZELKORN, FLORENCE: Some adaptations of basic concepts and principles for casework practice in a rehabilitation setting. *Proceedings of the Workshop: Practice of Social Work in Rehabilitation.* Chicago, U. of Chicago, 1960, p. 115.

HOLLIS, FLORENCE: *Casework: A Psychosocial Therapy.* New York, Random, 1964, p. 243.

JAMES, ALICE: Roles and responsibilities of social work: A key to practice in rehabilitation. In *Proceedings of the Workshop: Practice of Social Work in Rehabilitation.* Chicago, U. of Chicago, 1960, pp. 132-138.

RICE, ELIZABETH P.: Medical and health services. In *Encyclopedia of Social Work,* New York, Nat. Assn. of Social Workers, 1965, p. 472.

WHITE, ESTHER: The body-image concept in rehabilitating severely handicapped patients. *Social Work, 6*(3):52, 1961.

Chapter XII

ROLE OF THE DIETITIAN

In view of the fact that rehabilitation of the stroke patient involves a comprehensive plan of care, nutrition must be given its proper emphasis. However, too frequently the dietitian is a forgotten member of the team. For many people the process of eating is so routine and habitual it is taken for granted. Also most individuals have controlled their own eating habits for years and consider themselves minor experts in the field. Food habits and eating patterns are profoundly influenced by culture, religion, and socioeconomic factors. Therefore it is impossible to talk of nutrition as if it were an isolated fact. As a team member the dietitian must promote nutrition as an integral part of daily living and insure consideration of its inclusion in the comprehensive plan of care.

Anticipation and prevention are considerably more desirable than the remedying of avoidable damage due to stroke. Nutrition can play an important role in prevention. Persons with atherosclerosis, hypertension, or diabetes are in the high risk group. Management of these underlying conditions includes diet.

There is almost unanimous agreement that weight control or correction of obesity is helpful in all of these conditions. With weight loss, blood pressure goes down even without excessive sodium restriction. A common observation has been that an increase in weight almost inevitably brings a concomitant increase in blood pressure. Diabetes is more easily controlled when the patient is not overweight. In atherosclerosis the effect of obesity per se on the disease is not entirely clear, but it is safe to assume that it would be wise to control weight.

The use of unsaturated fats in the diet is still controversial, although there is strong evidence that they may be helpful in delaying or reversing symptoms of artherosclerosis.

When a stroke occurs, specific and challenging nutritional problems suddenly manifest themselves. The consistency of the patient's food needs to be drastically altered and the patient's ability to feed himself may be reduced to nothing. What has happened before the stroke should not be ignored however. The stroke patient has spent a lifetime developing his food habits, and his nutritional status is the end result of all his previous experiences. Preexisting attitudes and habits regarding food can affect diet therapy and possibly the progress of the rehabilitation program itself.

It may be helpful to review some of the reasons why people eat the way they do and in particular the effect of illness on food intake. The social value of food is known to all. Eating is an act of friendship, a convivial fellowship enjoyed without any thought of nutritional adequacy. However, for the individual who lives alone, mealtime may cease to be a pleasure. In the genesis of food habits, loneliness or "aloneness" must never be discounted. The isolation and withdrawal experienced by many individuals in old age are often associated with a considerable reduction of food intake. The stroke patient may experience more than his share of isolation and withdrawal with its resultant effect on nutrition.

Eating may not be pleasant when the patient has poor motor skills and limited range of motion. Mechanical difficulties such as paralysis of the face or throat make eating messy and disagreeable. The patient may be left to eat by himself away from others. Since people's lives are set in families, this isolation may represent ostracism and loss of status. He may feel that he is no longer a member of his family unit or socially acceptable. All of this can affect the amount of food a patient will eat.

In his earlier attempts at feeding himself, a certain patient may prefer privacy. Drawing the curtain around his bed or closing the door to his room will insure the privacy desired. However as he progresses he should be encouraged, unless the idea is totally distasteful to him, to join others at mealtime. If his fellow diners are carefully selected, group dining can help boost his morale and appetite. His meal companions should be willing to expect and to overlook slow motion and untidiness.

Food can be an emotional outlet. Overeating is often a way of compensating for disappointments and frustrations. For the aging person, familiar eating habits may provide security against apprehension and potential dangers. He may cling to his old habits in an attempt to make time stand still and to hold back its ravages. The rigidly held attitudes and rituals associated with food and eating provide a stronghold in a changing world where there are few controllable elements.

With the onset of the stroke, the patient finds he is unable to continue eating in the way in which he has become accustomed. Initially he may have to be fed soft or semiliquid foods or even baby foods. A diet of this type can easily convey a sense of deprivation and infantile helplessness to the patient. It may lead to discouragement that may often be masked by anorexia.

Even though the foods must be strained, it may be helpful to serve them in their whole state whenever possible. For instance, carrots or asparagus tips can be mashed with a fork at the table or on the tray. Each food could be served separately rather than in a combination. An apathetic patient should not be asked whether or not he wants to eat, but rather which food he prefers having first. The patient should be allowed to make choices, and whenever possible his personal feeding rituals should be observed. He should be fed as he would ordinarily eat, using his usual rotation of food and drink. Although his decisions may be relatively unimportant, he should be allowed to express his choices as a responsible adult.

The illness itself has an effect on food intake. Regressive attitudes may manifest themselves and focus on food. The patient may desire or reject certain foods as a result of previous experiences or in a childish attempt to gain attention. Food for the stroke patient should be of a proper consistency so that it will be easier to eat and provide less frustrations. If the patient's appetite becomes finicky, the dietitian can plan a diet more fitting to the patient's taste.

If the foods with the greatest appeal to the patient are judiciously selected, the dietitian can make the diet acceptable as well as nutritionally adequate. It should be remembered that not only the adequacy, but the actual consumption of the diet is important. A periodic evaluation of the patient's dietary intake should be made, particularly when appetite and motivation may be lacking. As the patient progresses and his appetite improves, diet changes can be made accordingly. Attention should be focused on the individual rather than the disease. It is impossible to achieve maximal result from diet therapy if the psychic and social factors are ignored.

Negativism, personality changes, and anxiety are often observed in the stroke patient, and they may have a direct bearing on appetite and food consumption. If the patient suddenly appears irritable or uncooperative and refuses to eat, he should not be forced. The feeding process should be stopped and resumed later. It may be a temporary fit of temper that will pass if handled with patience and understanding.

The patient may lack endurance, and he may find that the act of eating is fatiguing. The most nourishing meal should be served earlier in the day when the patient is fresh after a night's rest and when the appetite may be better. Smaller, more frequent meals are indicated when appetite and vitality are lacking.

In his prestroke days, the patient may have been on a nutritionally inadequate diet. One of the reasons could have been economic. Meager incomes are not often stretched to include nutritionally adequate foods. Meats, fruits, and vegetables are expensive items, and often the person with little money for food prefers to buy the high starchy foods that are cheaper.

Physical changes which result in decreased metabolism or which modify the mechanical part of eating also influence dietary intake and its utilization. Poor teeth or the lack of them interfere greatly with the ability of the person to meet his nutritional needs. With advanced age and possibly with a disabling condition, some persons may find it difficult to get proper dental attention. If teeth are missing or if dentures fit poorly, an individual may find it necessary to avoid the foods which need chewing. Since bulk-forming foods and some protein foods need chewing, these are often omitted from the diet.

The constipation one finds in elderly patients may be due, in part at least, to the lack of bulk-forming foods in the diet. The muscle and tissue wasting which is sometimes noted in the elderly patient may not be entirely due to the aging process. Perhaps the body is not getting sufficient protein foods for tissue building and replenishment.

The patient may have been on a restricted diet. Most therapeutic diets are based on NRC recommendations. Too often the patient fails to comprehend dietary instructions completely and accurately or he may add refinements of his own which may not be compatible with good nutrition.

At the time of the stroke the patient may not show overt signs of malnutrition, but his nutritional status may be far below par. If an active rehabilitation program is to be planned, can the progress of the patient be expected to go as well as if he had been well nourished? Good nutrition becomes an important part of the treatment in an attempt to overcome any possible dietary deficiencies and to gain strength for the more strenuous aspects of the rehabilitation program.

The objectives of good nutrition are to build and repair tissues and to provide energy for all body activities. In illness, a state of good nutrition may assist in hastening recovery and in avoiding complications. Unless any nutritional deficiency is corrected or avoided, the patient may remain chronically ill although his condition has been brought under control. Nutritional deficiencies can cause symptoms so vague and nonspecific that they are often overlooked or their underlying causes go unsuspected. When the patient is apathetic, depressed and anorexic, attention should be given to his nutrition. Is he eating what he should? If not, why not?

In the course of the rehabilitation program the patient may be called upon to use certain of his muscles in a more strenuous manner than he had been accustomed to doing. Something as simple as rolling over in bed or sitting up from a prone position may require much strength and effort from the patient. Muscle strengthening therefore is necessary for the success of the rehabilitation program. Eating body-building foods will not bring about an overnight change, but it can guard against a gradual weakening of the patient and possible retrogression.

The prime body-building food is protein, and special attention should be given to protein intake. The body does not store protein the same way fat is stored. The proteins in the liver, pancreas, blood plasma, kidney, and intestinal wall have a high rate of turnover, while the rate of turnover in the muscle, skin, bone, lung, and brain is lower. Even though the rate of turnover is slow in muscle mass there is a significant amount of protein mobilized. The proteins of some tissues may be "loaned" to other tissues where the need may be more urgent. If the diet does not supply sufficient protein, body muscles may supply protein needs. As a result, damage occurs in the form of muscle wasting and general weakness. When the wasted muscles can no longer supply the necessary protein, the levels of blood protein will fall with a resulting loss of resistance to injury and infection. In the presence of protein deficiency the patient is also more likely to develop edema and shock. Decubiti may develop even where there are no signs of failure in nursing techniques.

With extensive immobility of all or parts of the body, there can be a rapid breakdown and loss of protein. This can occur within a few days after injury or illness. Breakdown of protein may be indicated by nitrogen or potassium excretion in the urine or lowered protein levels in the blood. A weight loss of ten pounds or more in an adult occurring in a period of a few days or weeks is an excellent indication of protein loss.

To overcome protein deficiency, protein in the diet should range from 100 to 150 gm. Total calories must also be adequate. When calories are inadequate, the protein is deaminized and transformed into carbohydrates to provide energy. If protein intake must be increased, it should be gradual and not too excessive. An excess of protein may increase blood urea nitrogen to dangerous levels. To guard against any deficiency an observation of the actual protein consumed each day should be standard routine.

Arteriosclerosis may retard the utilization of food. Where arteriosclerotic narrowing in the arteries impairs circulation, the rate and volume of the blood flow is diminished. When the quantity of blood is decreased, the quality of the diet assumes greater significance than in a younger person whose more readily accelerated flow can compensate for deficiencies.

Meals should be planned with more than nutritional adequacy

in mind. The feeding process can be an important adjunct to other forms of therapy. Speech requires the use of certain facial and throat muscles which are also needed in eating. Working with the speech therapist, the dietitian can include foods in the diet which would aid speech therapy. Bowel and urinary training require a regularity of the diet and fluid intake which the dietitian can assist the nurse in planning. Even physical therapy and occupational therapy can be helped by including finger foods and other types of foods which necessitate the use of specific muscles and reflexes. Here again a close working relationship is needed among the members of the team.

A strong patient education unit should be part of any rehabilitation program. The patient and his family need to know as much as possible about the patient's condition and to understand the reasons for the various types of therapy. With adequate knowledge the patient and his family can assume their share of responsibility in the rehabilitation program. The dietitian can make great contributions through patient and family education. His activities include developing nutrition teaching aids and providing diet counseling.

More than one diet instruction is often needed. To provide follow-up and to extend nutrition services the dietitian must often depend on other members of the team whose contacts with the patient are more direct and continuous. Through in-service programs and consultations the dietitian can help his fellow workers to integrate nutrition into their own programs thereby maintaining an efficient and effective continuity of dietary care. This dietary care will take into consideration the level of severity of the patient's condition and the special circumstances, physical, social, or economic, attendant to the situation.

Adequate diet instruction cannot be provided unless one knows about previous food patterns, economic status, home conditions, and shopping facilities. To attempt diet counseling without this information is almost a total waste. By assisting in the assessment of home and family conditions the dietitian can make recommendations which will help make the diet prescriptions more realistic and the goals more readily obtainable.

Just as physical accomplishments may regress once the patient goes home, so may dietary planning. Nutrition can be a great problem especially when the patient has physical limitations and when the diet still needs some modification.

There are several community programs which are helping to meet the nutritional needs of the patient in the community. One of these is Meals-on-Wheels. Hot meals are prepared and delivered to recipients who are unable to shop for food or unable to prepare adequate meals. It is not necessary for a person to be bedridden to receive this service. The fees are usually based on ability to pay. These programs may employ paid help, but usually they are dependent on volunteers. Sponsorship may be varied; it might be sponsored by a senior citizens council, a church group, a health department or a service club. The meals are usually planned by trained dietitians. The meals may also include special diets. In all programs, the recipients receive one hot meal per day. Some programs also deliver cold foods sufficient for one or two meals. These foods may consist of sandwiches and fruit for a future lunch or supper, or a cold cereal and fruit for breakfast.

A second service that is quite popular is the Homemaker or Home Health Aide Service. The trained Homemaker or Home Health Aide goes into the home to help maintain family routine and to preserve the integrity of the family unit in time of stress. Nutrition teaching is done in a subtle way via nutritious meals prepared by the trained Homemaker or Home Health Aide. Help in meal planning and food purchasing are also a part of this service. Nutrition consultation is usually available to the service.

A third program is the Home Care Program. It may be based either in a hospital or in a community or in a local health department. In a hospital Home Care program, the hospital dietitian or the outpatient clinic dietitian may provide for nutrition consultation. In a community or local health department, the local or state health department nutritionist functions as a consultant. The nutritionist works closely with other key members of the Home Care team. He participates in in-service staff education and in the evaluation of the patient's progress. He functions mostly as a consultant and he usually visits only a small percentage of homes.

A recent service in many leading cities is Dial-A-Dietitian. Dial-A-Dietitian is a free telephone service offered to the community as a service of the state dietetic association. It is staffed by trained dietitians and nutritionists who have volunteered their services. The purpose of the program is to provide sound information on normal nutrition in an effort to combat the spread of diet misinformation. By providing authoritative answers to questions on normal nutrition, nutrient content of food, special diet recipes, chemical additives to food, food preparation, purchasing, and many other inquiries of this type, Dial-A-Dietitian is able to present the facts to the public. Dietary prescriptions and medical advice are not given, but the clients are referred to the family physician or appropriate agencies. Dial-A-Dietitian is simple for the public to use. The client needs only to dial a special number and ask his question. The answering service records the question and sends it to the dietitian who has volunteered to answer questions for that day. The dietitian telephones the client usually within forty-eight hours and gives him the answer to his question.

In certain low-income housing developments, Home Management programs have been started. The object of these programs is to teach better homemaking practices to residents in the housing developments. Each Home Management Aide works in individual homes on a one-to-one basis with the woman of the house. Cooking, cleaning, food purchasing, and sewing are some of the topics taught. Working with the handicapped or disabled person could be an area where the Home Management Aide might broaden her activities. Unlike the Homemaker services whose "primary function is the maintenance of household routine and the preservation or creation of wholesome family living in times of stress" through the presence and efforts of a trained Homemaker or Home Health Aide, the Home Management program is primarily an educational program. Its goal is self-improvement which will lead to improved household routines and the creation and promotion of wholesome and healthful family living. The Home Management program is geared to those who are physically able to perform household tasks, but it could include the physically handicapped. Work simplification techniques could be taught the stroke patient to enable him to function more effectively in his own home and to increase his independence. Under proper supervision the Home Management Aide could help provide follow-up at home of diet therapy and occupational therapy initiated in the hospital.

In general the principles of nutritional therapy can be summarized as follows:

There should be moderation in intake. It should be remembered that excess calories contribute to malnutrition just as much as deficiencies. There should be a liberal fluid intake. Balance in the dietary intake is important. The therapeutic diet is a modified normal diet and nutritional deficiencies concomitant with disease must be watched for and managed. The diet must be psychologically acceptable to the patient. There must be an attempt to individualize the diet as much as possible. It must be remembered that there are variations in physiological requirements, tolerance, and capacities. General dietary rules must be individually modified more often than not with attention focused on the individual rather than the disease.

As a member of the rehabilitation team the nutritionist should participate actively in the planning conference and in the periodic review of the patient's condition.

The nutritionist can help determine the nutritional objectives, and it should be his function to keep other team members alerted to the changing dietary needs of the patient. It is only when adequate attention is paid to the nutritional needs of the stroke patient that it can be said that truly total care is being given to the patient.

SUGGESTED READINGS

Allbrink, Margaret: Diet and cardiovascular disease. *J Amer Diet Assoc,* 46:26, 1965.

Brown, Helen, and Farrand, Marilyn: Pitfalls in constructing a fat-controlled diet. *J Amer Diet Assoc,* 49:303, 1966.

Campbell, Donald E.: Influence of diet and physical activity on blood serum cholesterol of young men. *Amer J Clin Nutr,* 18:79, 1966.

Fats in food and diet, A fact sheet for leaders. U. S. Department of Agriculture, Agricultural Research Service, March, 1966.

Heart Disease, The Tangled Web of Evidence. Special Report. *Chem Engin News,* 43:130, 1965.

MAY, ELIZABETH ECKHARDT; WAGGONER, NEVA R., AND BOETTKE, ELEANOR M.: *Homemaking for the Handicapped.* New York, Dodd, 1966.

OVERS, ROBERT P., AND BELKNAP, ELSTON: Educating stroke patient families. *J Chronic Dis, 20:45,* 1967.

SEBRELL, W. H., JR.: Changing concepts of malnutrition. *Amer J Clin Nutr,*

STEIDLE, ROSE E., AND BRATTON, ESTHER CREW: *Work in the Home.* New York, Wiley, 1968.

20:653, 1967.

ZUKEL, MARJORIE: Fat-controlled diets. *Amer J Clin Nutr, 16:270,* 1965.

Chapter XIII

ROLE OF CONSULTANTS

THE PSYCHOLOGIST

T HE PSYCHOLOGIST'S FUNCTION in a stroke rehabilitation setting coordinates with those of other medical and paramedical staff, at every step in the patient's progress from admission to discharge. This begins with the assessment process, leading to the setting of goals and making of specific treatment recommendations. Once treatment is under way, the psychologist serves as a consultant in problems of patient motivation, management of emotional problems, and may take the role of therapist with groups or individual patients. He often engages in research or consults in research design. The psychologist relates in the following manner with the other members of the rehabilitation team in carrying out these functions.

Assessment

The unique and specialized function of the psychologist is in the evaluation of mental abilities and personality traits as they stand after injury to the brain. The range of psychological after-effects of stroke or other brain injury causing hemiplegia is enormous. At one extreme, the hemiplegic may be absolutely intact in language and mental efficiency and respond to his handicap as though it were a purely orthopedic problem. At the other extreme, the hemiplegic may be not only speechless, but reduced intellectually to the performance of the minimum routines of self-care.

Aside from determination of an overall *level* of mental function, the psychologist must be prepared to look for and identify a variety of specific deficits in complex perceptual and motor skills. Among these deficits are the loss of recall of purposeful movements (apraxia), left-right confusion, neglect of stimuli on the same side of space as the paralysis, and of course, aphasic defects of oral expression, comprehension, reading, and writing. Such specific deficits may appear in a context of well-preserved general intelligence. They have very distinct implications in terms of ultimate rehabilitation goals and in terms of the treatment methods which may prove effective. Acquaintance with the area of psychological after-effects of brain injury is a sub-specialty among clinical psychologists and is often referred to as "neuropsychology." There is some overlap between this type of a psychological assessment and a neurologist's examination, with respect to the examination of mental status and specific perceptual motor deficits.

Beyond the case study of the patient's mental capacities, the psychologist devotes himself to evaluating the personality characteristics and emotional problems which must be taken into account. This assessment consists in part of a reconstruction of the premorbid personality from the case history and from current behavior. In part, it consists of interpretation of current behavior and of the results of projective personality tests. We know that radical "changes of personality" sometimes occur with brain injury. A reactive depression, reversible with appropriate management, may be confused with the relatively irreversible apathy which sometimes accompanies brain injury. Suspiciousness and irascibility may be seen in highly controlling individuals who are unable to tolerate the dependent role into which they are thrust. On the other hand, irascibility may be a manifestation of disinhibition of emotional controls and signal a profound deterioration in the personality. These examples illustrate the type of issues which may be resolved as the psychologist aids with interpreting the observed surface behavior.

The psychologist may collaborate specifically with the physician-in-charge in the preliminary screening evaluation of certain applicants. This may, for example, be the case when a patient who comes principally because he has aphasic and intellectual problems is presented as a candidate for admission to the program. In such a case, the psychologist and the speech therapist may jointly carry out a preadmission screening evaluation to assess the capacity of the patient to profit from retraining, both in terms of motivation and in terms of the preservation of basic perceptual and comprehension skills.

The psychologist brings before the physician-in-charge the salient findings which bear on the patient's ability to profit from the rehabilitation program. For example, a patient, though hemiplegic and densely aphasic, may be virtually intact in his reasoning powers, perceptual motor skills, and memory. Another individual, although superficially alert, may give test evidence of massive irreversible deficits in all modes of intellectual expression.

Goal Setting and Recommendations

Depending on the organizational structure of the rehabilitation center, the psychologist's findings may be brought into the treatment picture through various possible channels, generally both by discussion at a staff conference and by individual consultations with the rehabilitation specialists whose work is influenced by psychological findings. Taking the example of the staff conference as the main formal channel of information exchange, the psychologist on summarizing his findings, interprets their significance for each aspect of the rehabilitation program, as well as for the overall program. For example, the physical and occupational therapists may learn that a patient's apraxia constitutes an immediate objective of treatment as well as a limitation on the mode of approach. The patient may be capable of learning movements by imitation, but not be capable of performing to command in spite of all the sympathetic urging the therapist may summon. The level of intellectual function and the presence of possible defects in visual spatial skills has particular bearing on the complexity of the activity chosen in occupational or manual arts therapy.

The contribution of the clinical psychologist is particularly relevant to the job of the vocational rehabilitation counselor. The vocational counselor may employ specialized interest and aptitude tests, but his own choice of test will be influenced by the overall rehabilitation outlook outlined by the psychological assessment. The personality evaluation is of critical importance in determining the suitability of the patient for a training assignment and for the demands of a particular type of work setting. Thus, repeated consultation during the period of the patient's progress is to be expected between the psychologist and vocational specialist.

The social worker interacts collaboratively with the clinical psychologist both at the point of initial assessment and during the extended period when proper management is so important to maintaining the patient's motivation. Information obtained from the family on the patient's premorbid personality and abilities is to be put alongside the psychological test data in reconstructing the picture of the individual as he was premorbidly. Such a full understanding of the patient's background is valuable for the entire rehabilitation staff. It helps them to look on him and behave towards him in a manner coherent with his premorbid self-concept.

The psychologist contributes to the social worker's clear understanding of the patient's current mental functioning which in turn, the social worker interprets to the patient's family. The understanding and supportive attitude of the family is important to the patient's morale and may be critical in deciding whether he eventually returns to his family or to a nursing home.

Treatment

When a person is deeply preoccupied with unsolved underlying emotional problems he may be unable to attend to the work at hand as the symptoms of his preoccupation crop up in one form or another. Most hemiplegic patients are prey to emotional disturbances due to their physical disability and to the effect of this handicap on their interpersonal relationships. They have suffered a loss of the sense of bodily integrity, a loss which some individuals quite normally experience with depression, others as a challenge to counteraction, and others as a signal for regression to childishly passive and irresponsible behavior. This handicap confronts them with unaccustomed and unwelcome changes in family demands and expectations. Perhaps there is unspoken resentment and disappointment from the wife towards a husband who has let her down by becoming sick; perhaps there is also the corresponding feeling on the part of the hemiplegic patient. He may see the entire rehabilitation program as predicated on his accepting a new physical status and a new social and occupational role. His need to deny this reality demand may be expressed in his active or passive resistance to the program. The listing of the varieties of specific disturbances can go on endlessly, depending on the premorbid personality of the patient, on the family's attitude, and the real nature of the imposed disabilities. Whatever the specific form of any individual's symptoms of emotional disorders, these patients have problems in common which can profitably be taken up by patients meeting together in therapeutic discussion groups. Most clinical psychologists have had training and experience in the leadership of such groups. The technique of coleaders or a leader-observer team provides a means for another staff person such as the social worker or rehabilitation nurse to share in this function and develop the techniques for therapy-group leadership. In some cases individual psychotherapy may be more effective than group therapy. The consulting psychiatrist may be available to treat one or more such patients. More often his consultation takes the form of periodic review and supervision of the therapeutic management of the patients being seen by the psychologist or social worker.

Not all the emotional difficulties of the hemiplegic patient need be attacked by psychotherapy. Supportive counseling from the psychologist or help from him in understanding a patient's behavior may be valuable in tiding any of the therapy specialists through a difficult period with a patient who may be depressed, apathetic, rebellious, etc. As an expert on behavior who is somewhat more objective and detached with respect to the interactions with the patient in rehabilitation therapy, the psychologist is the natural resource person for informal consultation.

Research

There are many potential lines for systematic investigation in relation to the treatment of the hemiplegic patient. Unplanned studies usually result in reports which contribute nothing to the advancement of knowledge about effective treatment. Because of his specific training in research methods, statistics, and the logic of scientific investigation, the psychologist is often used as a consultant not only in research areas bordering on psychology, but in other areas which are not usually regarded as psychological. The role of the research consultant is first to help the investigator reframe his question in terms which can be experimentally tested; second, to set up the conditions of experimental observation so that the logic of the experiment requires that different results lead to specifically different inferences. He may also set up the statistical analysis of the data so as to be able to discriminate which results could not be obtained by chance.

The foregoing description of the functions of a clinical psychologist is somewhat overdrawn in that one individual would probably be unable fully to carry out all the suggested activities. Depending on the orientation of the rehabilitation center, one or the other of these activities may be highlighted and others omitted.

THE PSYCHIATRIST

The public views the psychiatrist as a person who works with patients who are physically sound, but whose inner problems keep them from making a satisfactory adjustment. Today, more and more psychiatrists are working in general hospitals and treating people who have physical handicaps, and special reactions to medical illness and surgical treatment. The psychiatrist has come to share responsibility for the overall management of organically damaged patients along with the other professionals involved in their care. Clinical psychologists, neurologists, internists, surgeons, and social workers have been traditionally involved in studying and helping patients who have had cerebrovascular accidents. In the case of stroke patients the psychiatric consultations are often focused on the patient who is particularly difficult or uncooperative in the rehabilitation program. It is notable that rehabilitation units which function efficiently with high morale tend to require less psychiatric consultation. This is due to the obvious fact that "good medicine" has always involved an awareness of the patient as a person, as a unique individual with a special style and special resources; and rehabilitation teams which work well do so because they handle emotional upheavals with clear leadership and a unified management of the environment. This resolves many problems which might otherwise blossom into serious psychiatric upsets. This also explains the seeming paradox that units with great effectiveness and enthusiam are often very psychologically aware but do not often need psychiatric consultation; this awareness leads to more sensitive handling of patients and fewer psychiatric emergencies. Often enough, the call for a psychiatric consultant results from a sense of failure on the part of the staff when they cannot comprehend, sympathize with, or control the behavior of a patient. The staff often wants to hand over the confused, agitated stroke patient who is incoherent. If the psychiatrist is successful in his work he can make suggestions about medication, environmental manipulation, and ways of communicating with the patient which will bridge the confusion of the brain-damaged disturbed patient and the sense of defeat on the part of the staff so they can again focus on the rehabilitation plan. Psychotherapy is usually short-term adjunct therapy aimed at easing the behavioral sabotage of the overall rehabilitation. To be most helpful the psychiatrist should share the rehabilitation philosophy of the group. He needs to be able to clarify the meaning of behavior in aphasic, brain-injured, and somewhat disoriented patients who also have emotional upsets, and to be able to present the explanations in words that help the staff to better accept troublesome responses and attitudes in patients.

Basic Reactions to Illness

Anxiety, regression, and depression are the three basic reactions seen in most illnesses. Anxiety is usually defined as a sense of dread and expectation that something damaging is about to happen. This is distinguished from fear and expectation of being harmed which occurs in response to clear physical danger. In contrast, anxiety refers to an emotion evolving within the patient. It is important to note that anxiety is a quality found in all individuals as a basic reaction and does not imply disease by its existence, but refers to an internal sense that something is going to happen. One of the most common examples is the sensation that students have before exams when the intensity of their emotion clearly transcends the actual threat of the examination. With stroke patients there is frequently a tremendous upsurge of this affect when they have to begin to walk. It seems clear that the concern that they express goes beyond the risk of tumbling down when they walk; they treat the event and the challenge of having to ambulate as almost a life or death matter. Similarly, when patients are about to be discharged and have to take over responsibility they frequently show an increase in anxiety. For all objectively limited stroke patients there is considerable concern arising from doubt about what they can do; they are worried about what will happen to them in an emergency; they are worried about losing control of their bodies; they are worried about appearing foolish or being too noticeable in public; all of these situations may stir up unpleasant dread in the patient.

Another kindred reaction to illness is regression; this is the return to patterns of behavior which are appropriate to an earlier age. For the child, bedwetting, infantile speech, and whining are among the commonest types of regression seen in the hospital. With adults who have had strokes, their tremendous helplessness forces upon them regressive behavior. They must be washed, they need to be helped to stand, to clothe themselves, to be fed; for self-sufficient individuals this change of status is both unpleasant and frightening and also inevitable. For patients to fight too strongly against any regression may in itself present problems. If a patient who is unprepared insists on helping himself and refuses to take assistance at appropriate times he can create enormous problems for himself. There are other patients who float into the situation of being totally cared for by others with such zeal that they present difficulties when they have to be pressed toward self-sufficiency.

Depression is a universal experience. People lose hope; many feel they are being punished and that the future is bleak. They look backward at past joys. In minor illnesses such as the flu, or a cold, people will often complain, seem irritable and grouchy and show rather simple forms of the depression. They think back to the preceding week when they felt healthy. Older, disabled people turn to the more distant past. Stroke patients may mask the demonstration of their emotions, and if they are older people some of the sadness of aging and loneliness may shade over into a kind of apathy, an apparent lack of deep feeling. Nonetheless, it is important to note that depression characterizes these sick people and is an appropriate and universal part of the situation. This gentle, omnipresent mood is an antagonist against which the staff in the rehabilitation unit must constantly struggle. Depressed stroke patients muse about their own previous lives; they daydream, and they suffer from the loss of hope they attribute to their vascular accidents.

Psychic Energy

All individuals in the course of their daily lives are aware of variations in physical energy. However, it is only with the physically ill, the emotionally disturbed or the aged that these variations in energy become central problems. Elderly people take a good deal of time planning how much they can do to handle the fatigue that they feel. This is part of the process of aging. Along with the general deterioration that underlies the aging process is a series of metabolic changes that diminishes the energy reserve. This is shown in the psychological sphere in a variety of ways: the individual has diminished power of concentration, greater disability in absorbing unfamiliar information, and a decrement in the recall of previously learned information. These features in the alien environment of the hospital all work against the satisfactory adaptation of the patient to the hospital. The combination of diminished energy and a sense of being unable to cope with the surroundings leads to a profound sense of helplessness.

In all people there are rhythms of hope, optimism, discouragement and anticipation. By its very nature, depression involves looking backward instead of forward; people tend to look at the past and concentrate on the misdeeds or omissions of that period. Old age is a time of looking backward, and this is reenforced by hospitalization and disability. The typical old person in or out of the hospital is surrounded by pictures of departed relatives, children, and mementoes of the past.

It is important to note that the staff itself undergoes rhythmic changes of morale and that these influence patient performance and behavior. Staff members are involved in very specific goals of therapy and may incorrectly assume that the stroke patient, particularly the elderly one, shares the goal. In reality, such patients are often preoccupied, inattentive, and depleted. Strokes usually occur in the older population already struggling with geriatric problems. The diminution of intellectual capacities particularly in areas involving speed, memory, and adaptability may be strikingly increased by a vascular accident. Emotional resilience may be greatly limited in old or young stroke patients. It is important to note that in the aging process in general and in reactions to stroke, the personality impairment or the deterioration of competence do not bear a direct relation to the amount of brain damage. Some elderly people with marked arteriosclerosis and many senile plaques function well while others with more intact tissue are reduced to minimal functioning. The drop in mental ability is very much related to basic personality. The young stroke patient is more likely to be cut off in the prime of life, in the midstream of uncompleted tasks, and to suffer from emotional shock, active horror about himself, and a frustrated depressive response to being thwarted in his life course. The older person may have had small strokes and time to prepare himself for decrements in ability. However, the ongoing pattern of aging produces restriction of the personality and brittle responses. For many older people, staying home in the evening, driving for short periods, limiting their travels to familiar places, all occur without noticeable change in their personality. If they are not called upon to learn new things or to be very specific about old information they do not show much loss. But when suddenly placed in a new environment, like the hospital, or when they sustain a small stroke, it may be enough to sharply expose already poorly functioning mental faculties. Aldridge points out that the mental hygiene of old age begins in childhood and that an adult who has developed superior adaptive capacity can adapt to new areas or productivity when the physical and economic constrictions of old age shut off his previous outlets. Naturally, the rehabilitation staff cannot remake the individual, but the more informed the staff members are about the special interests and accomplishments of each patient, the more skillfully they can encourage the stroke patient to get back to the things that interest him and to utilize the faculties that remain. It is also wise for the professional to know when he is weary and more likely to be surly and bring forth the least competent responses from the brain-injured individual.

Dependency is harder for young stroke patients to tolerate. The older patient has gradually shifted to ineffectualness, to partial reliance on others, and then to greater reliance on others whether relatives, friends, or social agencies. The younger person takes pride in his self-sufficiency and does not leap at the opportunity to have basic functions cared for by others. Unquestionably some dependent individuals slip readily into the patient role without any difficulty, and they may later become problems when they have to be wedged loose from their beds to walk and to take an active part in the rehabilitation process. For some people the disaster of a cerebrovascular accident produces a long period of dazed, uncomprehending inactivity; this shocklike condition can tail off into apathy and depression. Neurotic depression may intermingle with a depressive reaction to disaster. The loss of perception that a stroke may entail; poorer vision; scotomas; changes in space, heat and touch perception, may all add to the patient's feeling of incompetence and helplessness.

Hospitalization presents a major stress for any individual. Institutions often have definite atmospheres and attitudes toward chronic patients. The best-run hospitals are not as pleasant to live in as a modest home; they cannot be individualized that much. An institution which cares for the whole life of an individual inevitably produces dysculturation, the sense of loss of the interplay of events in the larger society. The stroke patient brings a less adaptable personality to this new, unfamiliar bustling environment. He brings with him a personal way of reacting which may be more hostile, more childlike, more controlling, or more full of idiosyncracies because of the stroke. Elderly people are notorious for concern about their bowels, about constipation, and they are notably grumpy and hypochondriacal. All of the individual sensitivities are likely to be exposed when privacy is absent, and dressing and undressing, and toilet are accomplished in a semipublic way albeit in a kindly manner. For the average person there is a certain way that his life space is organized, his room, his clothes, his toothbrush all have a pattern at home which is not possible in the hospital. The less elastic the person, the harder it is to make all of these adjustments. More familiar things from his home (pictures, etc.) help keep his orientation clear.

Patients with strokes often feel they are stigmatized. Goffman points out that stigma is used in medicine to refer to "bodily signs of physical disorders," but is applied more to the disgrace that is felt about defects than to the bodily evidence of the disorder. He describes how the social image or identity of individuals is defined by the ways people expect to treat each other, and the ways they are treated. The stroke patient has a deep sense of what society expects from the normal person, and feels a sense of what others see as his deficiency, inevitably causing him to see that he does fall short of what he ought to be. And this leads to a sense of shame, which is often not spoken, but nevertheless remains deeply felt in spite of the best public education about illness. So deeply embedded in people is the idea of the biblical "Lord, why hast thou foresaken me?" that when illness strikes, the individual often feels he has done something wrong to provoke it. Recriminations are most defined in individuals who had their strokes while engaged in some exertion such as sports, straining at stool, or sexual intercourse. This fosters the feeling that if the patient had *just not* done that act he would have escaped his particular fate. This is unsaid by the patients, but often involves a wish to hide themselves or their paretic limbs which has to be overcome by the physical therapist and the family.

Special Syndromes

A number of psychiatric studies of illness have worked out reaction profiles for different kinds of people. Nemiah has described how individuals who have always appeared vigorously independent and assertive may suddenly become whining, inconsolable, and cringing, because the facade of aggressiveness was a flimsy cover for a deeper attitude of dependency. For such patients it is important to understand the factors on the ward which may encourage infantilism in the particular patient. The consultant should be able to demarcate the limitations of the stroke patient's psychic resources which may be obstacles to successful rehabilitation. The staff members may have disagreements between them about the handling of patients. Stanton and Schwartz have explicated some of the ways in which underlying differences of opinion about patients may lead to poor management of patients, and upset responses in the patients. The psychiatrist can often be helpful in a sense in dissolving these covert conflicts. To do this he needs to be familiar with the jargon of the different workers and their special styles of working. This aspect has been stressed so often that some writers feel the best use of time might be for the psychiatrist to study the personalities of people going into rehabilitation work to find out which attitudes and personality patterns are most suited to the work. The many patients handled by each physical therapist, nurse, rehabilitation counselor, and social worker are vast and their helpfulness enormous. However, the damage and suffering that can be wrought by a disturbed professional worker in these fields is also immense. The psychiatric consultant may be useful in untangling some of the staff conflict and leading particular personnel members to a better awareness of their own conflicts and how these are manifested with patients.

Patients with similar disabilities can often work in groups for mutual help; these groups may be run by psychologists or social workers and can sometimes involve the stroke patients and their families, joining together to help advance the treatment plan. Psychiatrists can participate directly in some of these group approaches, or they can serve in a supervisory function.

The role of the psychiatrist clearly involves his acting as a relay for information. He needs to be careful about avoiding upset in these patients in the course of psychological probing. The aphasic patient who has feelings he cannot express will often harbor fears of being insane, and the manner of referral and its handling by the consultant should bring out this concern if it exists in order to allay it. The best approach is the most simple and direct one which tells the patient why he is being seen and makes clear that it is part of the therapy and not the beginning of a "dumping" procedure.

Suicide

Stengel points out that suicide rates have been found to be positively correlated to male sex, increasing age, widowhood, single and divorced state, childlessness, high density of population, residence in big towns, a high standard of living, economic crisis, alcohol consumption, history of broken home in childhood, mental disorder, and physical illness. It is clear that all of these factors either increase the isolation of the individual or produce a diminished ability to relate to others. Nonetheless, a well-run rehabilitation service does not usually have a high incidence of suicide threats or actual suicides. There are several reasons for this: First, the emotional energies of people who have had strokes are depleted and the residual emotional forces are involved in managing to live with what has happened. This seems to act against making a plan for terminating life. Secondly, the stroke patient is also very much amenable to the reassurances of the staff that living will be worthwhile even if he is not completely healthy. Thirdly, the physical disability also rules out some of the most likely methods of self-destruction. However, the best help in this really comes from the milieu when it provides forward-looking therapists who reach out to the patient and redirect him toward a useful existence and a higher level of functioning.

The threat of suicide cannot be totally ignored. Recent studies indicate that the majority of suicidal individuals make clear their intentions verbally and in writing well before they make any attempt. Hence the staff members should be alert to complaints which involve a statement of suicidal attempt. A history of previous suicidal attempts is a serious warning. If the patient accuses himself and seems to feel guilty about what he has done to his family and seems full of tension and anxiety this would be cause for alarm about such a possibility. If there is a family history of suicide or the recent suicide of a friend or significant person, it may also suggest the possibility to an individual. It is worth noting that when a patient is in a phase of recovering from a deep or lethargic depression he may be more likely to do something dangerous to himself. Patients who are almost stuporous with depression are usually unable to perform a self-destructive act. When they begin to loosen up in their frozen emotional state they may abruptly harm themselves. In dealing with any of these patients the most helpful attitude to take is one of direct sympathetic questioning. If a patient seems to be talking about harming himself, it's worth asking if this is what he has in mind so that help can be brought immediately. The responsibility of assessing a suicidal patient should properly be given to a psychiatric consultant if there is any question about the patient's symptoms or complaints.

Promoting Better Motivation

This may be interpreted as meaning an atmosphere aimed at progress for all patients. Ramona Todd has described a four-step approach to help attack the isolation of elderly patients. She describes first the formation of a one-to-one relationship between a staff member and a patient, then the introduction of another person, a "weaker individual . . . with more needs whom our patient can help, thus coming to feel needed." This also helps the weaker patient directly. She then advises placing these people into groups for therapy, and the use of this group by its leader to press for the reintegration of the patient into the community. This type of approach has much to recommend it for younger patients with strokes, as well as for the elderly. These patients, as all people, need a sense of being worthwhile. They have enormous concrete evidence in their symptomatology that their usefulness is over. For some, and this is particularly true of older normal people with a backlog of success in their lives, the patient merely needs to review his past successes and feel nurtured by thinking about what he was previously able to accomplish. This is similar to sitting and looking over one's mementoes, a rather general human experience. But for many aging or disabled individuals there is the large emotional hazard that they will be confronted with all they *did not do,* and with the lost opportunities for accomplishment and for pleasurable experiences which are not unobtainable.

The staff needs to be able to pick up clues from relatively inarticulate patients about what things really gave them a sense of worth, the ability to crochet, to fix a car, or the obvious universals of having had fine children and having supported a family. Finding bridges between the limited activities of the patients and the sense of competence from the past is what is needed. With younger patients, the amount of rage, frustration, and immediate sadness is greater. And it is less harmful in the long run to let these patients openly vent their feelings. It is less exhausting than in older people and provides a needed relief. Often, a young male who cries may need to be comforted about the reasonableness of his tears instead of shamed for breaking down and being unmanly.

Auxiliary Use of Drugs

People are the most effective therapeutic instruments with post cerebrovascular accident patients. Drugs can be very helpful, but they should be viewed in their proper role. Often, when a brain-damaged individual gets more attention, along with a new drug, it is the attention that is therapeutic, though the drug may get the credit. The assessment of psychologically active drugs remain a problem for this reason, though it is clear that the medications that are used in rehabilitation programs should be used as part of the overall approach, administered by the regular personnel and not generally by the consultant.

The most common problems with this group of patients are agitation, confusion, sleep disturbance, emotional lability, and depression. Because of the poorer absorption and diminished rate of excretion in some of these patients, along with the notorious decrease in the ability to hold ideas together, drugs may have quite unreliable results. It is often hard to elicit from aphasic patients a sense of feeling better, so that a trend toward lower dosages, scrupulous observation of verbal and motor responses to medication, and the use of as few medications as possible at the same time to avoid confusion about effects is important.

The variety of agents gaining current favor is enormous, but here only a few need be mentioned, basically under the heading of calming agents or energizing medications.

Calming Agents

Benadryl® (diphenhydramine HCL, Parke-Davis) in 25 mg capsules, is an old reliable antihistaminic. This quality makes it safer, but its long action and its quieting influence is a considerable help in calming elderly people who are agitated and who cannot sleep. One capsule b.i.d. is often a considerable maintenance dosage.

Barbiturates are notable for their tendency to produce disintegration of mental functioning in the brain-injured, the senile, and in children, with a paradoxical liberation of disorganized energy, and are not recommended.

Meprobamate (Equanil®, Miltown®) 400 mg tablets. Provides a mild tranquilizer with few side effects, a very low toxicity, and a wide range of dosage, and can be given up to 2000 mg daily. However, for the group of patients under discussion, sometimes it is hard to see any response.

Chlorpromazine (Thorazine®) 10 to 15 mg one to three times per day is among the most reliable and most widely tested drugs to relieve agitation in psychosis, or in organic brain conditions. It should be reserved for more severe states of confusion and delirium because of its occasional liver complications, extrapyramidal side effects and because it sometimes makes people who are concerned about their remaining intellectual functioning even more worried about what has happened to them.

Trifluoperazine (Stelazine®) 1 to 10 mg b.i.d. or t.i.d. is a related phenothiazine with a fluorine substitution in the chemistry which is believed to lower the liver toxicity, and appears useful in much smaller dosages. It would generally be used in the same situations. It may produce parkinsonian side effects.

Psychoactivators and Antidepressants

Amphetamine (Benzedrine®), *dextroamphetamine* (Dexedrine®), and *methamphetamine* (Desoxyn®) are all in tablet form and can be used in 2.5 to 10 mg dosages once a day to stimulate patients. They have the disadvantage of making many elderly patients feel apprehensive, and as they are also used for diminution of appetite, they may be problematical for patients who are also feeding problems. In small doses, for mildly dejected stroke patients, especially younger ones, they may add a sense of "zip" and boost morale. They should be used early in the day so as not to interfere with sleeping. They are not very helpful medications for major depressions.

Imipramine (Tofranil®) 10 to 25 mg b.i.d. or t.i.d. for clearly demarcated depressions. This medication requires seven to ten days to produce a reliable response, and frequently the intensified watchfulness of the doctors and nurses toward one of these patients may in itself produce improvement well before the drug is likely to do anything.

In the administration of any of these medications it is important to note the attitudes of the people doing the therapy. When patients are expected to improve emotionally, this often helps them to do so much more than an imperious expectation that a drug will do the job. At the same time, scrupulous interest about the dietary habits, the bowel functioning, and the ability to dress (especially in women), and to carry out the activities of daily living will all contribute significantly to overcoming the endemic problems of despair and inactivity in patients who have had cerebrovascular accidents.

Finally then, the role of the psychiatrist, as any other member of the rehabilitation team, is to facilitate participating in life on the part of the patient. To paraphrase Dr. Avery Weisman, "use what remains" and stimulate the remaining physical, emotional, and social faculties of the patient through a group effort by the rehabilitation staff.

The Vocational Counselor

To every stroke patient, male or female, who has been accustomed to working for a living or managing a household, comes the haunting fear that never again will it be possible to support self and/or family in the usual manner. The step from independence in self-management to adequate job performance is a major one. It becomes particularly complicated for stroke patients because many are left with significant impairments. However, the rehabilitation process is not complete unless all job potential is exploited.

The need for expert counseling has produced the professional vocational counselor who is able to provide many services to the stroke patient seeking return to employment. The vocational counselor is trained to review qualifications, to discover new skills, and to improve old ones. He makes a careful appraisal of the interest and aptitudes of the applicants, using standard psychological tests when they are appropriate. After consultation with the physician, he evaluates physical capacities and abilities. He then informs the applicant about current job opportunities and counsels him in a new field of endeavor. If necessary, he provides training or retraining to broaden or improve skills in a familiar field. If a number of stroke patients have common problems, group consultation techniques may be used. The counselor turns to selective placement when physical limitations require this to protect the patients, as well as the employer, from health and safety hazards.

As a team member in a rehabilitation center, a public rehabilitation agency counselor is valuable because of his knowledge of and control over the resources of the agency. These may be drawn upon to support a patient who is confined to the center during the early stages of a chronic disability. This may be a most decisive stage in the patient's total rehabilitation program.

Such a counselor should preferably have had at least two years of experience in the public agency serving a general client load. This will enable him to fully know his profession and feel confident in the practice of vocational rehabilitation counseling procedures.

The counselor functions by attending intake evaluation conferences as a team member. Patients at that time can usually be labelled as definitely unsuitable, definitely suitable, or potential. Further attention is then focused upon the latter two groups. Certain basic investigation is made such as previous employment, economic status, social status, educational level, special abilities, etc. The counselor then follows the prospective client in the progress he makes on the restorative program and at the proper time, in consultation with physician and staff, develops a vocational rehabilitation plan. The possibility of job placement, training, schooling, or retraining with a tentative time schedule and target date provides an effective antidote to the patients initial fear and despair.

This counselor must have enough control over the professional resources of his agency by himself or through his supervisor to demand performance in support of the plan as it develops. The agency should also provide support for the later stages of the plan as the restorative program ends and the patient returns to the community. At this time the patient is referred to the counselor in his own community for completion of the plan.

Vocational rehabilitation is a sound investment. In 1947 after World War II, 44,000 persons were vocationally rehabilitated and started to earn wages at a rate exceeding $70,000,000 a year. In 1949, they paid over $5,000,000 to the government in income taxes alone. Before rehabilitation, many of these patients were wholly or partially on local relief rolls, at an annual cost of $300 to $600 per case.

The vocational counselor must be positive in urging the need of his services to the doctors and other team members. In this way a total program will be insured.

REFERENCES

ALDRICH, C. KNIGHT: *Psychiatry for the Family Physician.* New York, McGraw, 1955.

ARIETI, SYLVANO (Ed.): *American Handbook of Psychiatry.* New York, Basic Books, 1959, vol. 2.

BELLAK, LEOPOLD: *Psychology of Physical Illness.* New York, Grune, 1952.

BERNSTEIN, N. R.: Management of patients with post-traumatic headache: Role of family physician and psychiatrist. *Headache, 4:*

BERNSTEIN, N. R.: The psychiatrist's role on the rehabilitation team. *J Rehab, 25:*22, 1959.

BONNER, C. D.: Medical progress, physical medicine and rehabilitation, *New Eng J Med, 271:*136, 1964.

GOFFMAN, ERVING: Stigma. *Notes on the Management of Spoiled Identity.* Englewood Cliffs, N. J., Prentice-Hall, 1963.

KLINE, NATHAN S., AND LEHMANN, HEINZ: *Handbook of Psychiatric Treatment in Medical Practice.* Philadelphia, Saunders, 1962.

NEMIAH, JOHN C.: Contribution of psychiatry to research in physical medicine and rehabilitation. *Arch Phys Med, 37:*6, 1956.

NEMIAH, JOHN C.: The psychiatrist and rehabilitation. *Arch Phys Med, 38:*3, 1957.

ODELL, C. E.: Employment and preretirement problems of older workers. II. Job counseling and placement services for persons over 40. *Geriatrics, 14:*518, 1959.

Rusk, H. A.: Rehabilitation: Report of council on physical medicine and rehabilitation. *JAMA, 140*:286, 1959.

Stanton, Alfred H., and Schwartz, Morris S.: *The Mental Hospital.* New York, Basic Books, 1954.

Stengel, Erwin: *Suicide and Attempted Suicide.* Baltimore, Penguin, 1964.

Todd, Ramona L.: Early treatment reverses symptoms of senility. *Hosp Comm Psych, 17*(6):40, 1966.

Chapter XIV

HOME EVALUATION PROGRAM

T HE REHABILITATION PROCESS for any patient, but especially the stroke patient who will be left with some significant degree of residual disability, cannot be completed without including the family and the home as a part of the comprehensive effort. The family is always initially involved with the rehabilitation process at the time of the admission of the patient to the program. Their next major involvement takes place when the patient has improved to the extent that a weekend visit at home is possible and safe.

The family at this time is invited into the center to spend an hour or two observing the patient's current performance as it relates to his activities of daily living, his general wheelchair or ambulatory mobility, his endurance, confidence, etc. The patient's capabilities are clearly outlined and demonstrated so that when he goes home he cannot regress to a stage of dependency by claiming that he is unable to perform certain routine procedures.

On the other hand, by seeing the patient actually perform routine tasks in an adequate and safe manner, the family becomes less apprehensive about letting the patient participate in the household activities. In this way, both patient and family come face to face with reality and reach a mutual understanding of what is to be expected during the first visit home. This visit is very important to the staff as well because it gives them a chance to assess the relationship of the patient to his family and family group, and at the end of the weekend the family or patient may bring back specific problems which the staff can work out before the next visit.

Of greater importance, however, is the home evaluation which is done just before the patient is permanently discharged to his home. By this time the staff knows the extent of residual physical disability with which the patient will have to contend. The residual disability may be in any one of a number of areas. The patient sometimes requires some assistance in the activities of daily living area or open wounds may need dressing. These involve the nurse. Problems may remain in mobility or transfer which would involve the physical therapist. The need to re-arrange a kitchen for function or safety would involve the occupa-tional therapist. The social worker may still be involved in adjustment problems as the patient returns to the family circle. If there is a speech or communication problem the speech therapist would be involved. In practice, any one or all of the therapists or social workers who have been involved with the patient during his hospitalization may desire to go on the home visit and evaluate the home as it relates to his field. In most instances the physical therapist is necessary and the physical and occupational therapists go together frequently as a team. In fewer instances, other combinations such as the nurse, physical therapist, and social worker, or physical therapist, speech thera-pist, and social worker, or nurse and occupational therapist, etc., make up the team for the evaluation. If there are students working with the patients in any of the departments, they are also included with the visiting team.

The appointment for the home evaluation is usually made through the social service office and at a time convenient to both family and hospital personnel. Usually the family comes to the hospital, picks up the patient and the team, and drives them to the home. They also return them to the hospital when the evaluation is completed. In other instances the therapists may utilize their own transportation or a taxi, but transporting patients in the staff's personal vehicles is avoided. If outside agencies such as the Visiting Nurse Association are going to be involved in the discharge planning members of these groups are also invited to be present at the time of the home evaluation. Once in the home each staff member investigates those features which fall under his field of operation. The physical therapist checks the staircases which the patient may have to navigate to get in and out of the house, as well as staircases he may have to go up and down in his daily routine within the house. The presence or need for railings on both sides of the stairs, the number and height of the stairs and any particular difficult turns which have to be executed are assessed. The status of large rugs and scatter rugs on the floor is keenly observed and the number and location of thresholds which fall in the path most commonly used by the patient, either ambulating or in a wheelchair is noted. The location or distribution of furniture in a room is studied so that it may be placed attractively but still functionally, thus eliminating hazards from the path of the patient. A great deal of attention is focused on the bathroom to see that the seat of the toilet is of the proper height, that appropriate grab bars or seat railings are installed, that safety strips are placed on the bottom of the bathtub, and appropriate grab bars and railings surround this so that the patient may be as independent as possible. A bathtub stool may be indicated, sturdy captain armchairs may be necessary, or a shower attachment may be suggested. The bedroom is assessed for the height of the bed, its firmness and appropriate placement in the room in relation to the side of the patient's disability. Dresser drawers and closet space are checked out in detail, so that clothing may be easily obtained and laid out for dressing.

The occupational therapist turns his attention to surveying the need for adaptive equipment necessary for the activities of daily living and also makes a detailed assessment of the kitchen and household situation. This is done especially for the female patient, but the male patient who can participate in household tasks may not only assist the female of the household, but also make it possible for her to become a wage earner if necessary. The arrangement of all commonly used utensils and pieces of household equipment becomes very important.

The social worker is a member of the team if difficult adjustment between family and patient is expected. He works closely with other agencies which may have to be involved in helping the patient make the best adjustment possible in the home. This is particularly necessary if the patient is going to the home of one of their own children where there are also small grandchildren and a son-in-law on the scene.

If the patient has any remaining nursing problems such as the dressing of healing pressure areas, the care of incontinence, or assistance in tub bathing, etc., this information would be transmitted to the family or to the Visiting Nurse Association if the services of the latter are deemed necessary.

The speech therapist would help to pinpoint any particular communication problems and assist the family in understanding how the patient expresses his needs by certain expressions, gestures, etc. At the end of the visit, concrete suggestions are made to the family in all perimeters. Those which have been made most frequently are listed in Table V.

After the home evaluation, the team returns to the center and submits their thoughts and suggestions on a standard form which is cleared through the social service department to the physician-in-charge (see Chart 9). The physician-in-charge reviews the form and recommendations, and following clarification of any questionable problems, sends a letter to the patient himself

TABLE V

MOST FREQUENTLY MADE RECOMMENDATIONS AT TIME OF HOME EVALUATION

1. Gate at top of stairs
2. Clothing adjustment
3. Chairs back to wall
4. Grab bar for toilet or safety frame
5. Washbowl stool
6. Bathtub seat
7. Grab bar for bathtub
8. Remove scatter rugs
9. Railings for stairs
10. Remove thresholds
11. Secure electric wiring
12. Hook back screen door
13. Moving of furniture for more wheelchair or walking space
14. Bed board
15. Lay out clothing
16. Wheelchair
17. Raised toilet seat
18. Shower attachment
19. New apartment on first floor
20. Pull-rope at end of bed
21. Sturdy chair for sitting
22. Remodeling of stairs
23. Urinal or bedpan at bedside during night
24. Supervision of aide
25. Low bed with railings
26. V. N. A. Supervision
27. Specific kitchen utensils
28. Change sleeping quarters to first floor
29. Bedside commode
30. Adjustment of electrical fixtures
31. Tighten knobs on bannister
32. Wax bureau drawers
33. Footstool for dressing
34. Removal of door and replacement of different type
35. Carrier basket
36. Bathtub mat
37. Ramp construction
38. Restraining strap when in wheelchair
39. Clothing in top bureau drawers
40. Supervision getting out of car
41. Drawer handles in center of drawer
42. Adjustment of venetian blind cords
43. Change of dwelling
44. Shoulder bag
45. Install overhead pulley
46. Night light
47. Do not drive automobile
48. Crutch hook
49. Remove casters from bed
50. Raise height of bed
51. Foam rubber cushion
52. Special number of rings at doorbell

or to a responsible family member thanking them for the privilege of making the visit, making them aware of some of the patient's remaining problems, and then listing the suggestions which the team would like to have the family consider incorporating into their home before the patient is discharged (see sample letter).

SAMPLE LETTER

NOVEMBER, 1967

DEAR

May I take this opportunity to thank you for allowing our team of therapists to visit your home in your behalf. We are happy that the time has come for you to be discharged, and we hope that you will focus on the realistic use of the abilities you have achieved. You must always think in terms of your own safety and not attempt to do things which may result in injury and regression.

We would like to make the following suggestions for your consideration:

1. As the bedroom is too narrow to admit the wheelchair, your bed should be placed as near to the door as possible.
2. A chair should be placed close to the bed for use in dressing and putting on the brace.
3. Removal of threshold going into the bathroom is necessary to allow the wheelchair to get into the room.
4. Rearrangement of furniture in the bathroom will be necessary to allow for wheelchair mobility.
5. A toilet seat frame should be in place.
6. A grab bar on the wall over the bathtub is necessary.
7. Adaptive equipment used in the kitchen should be clamped in place.
8. All scatter rugs should be removed.
9. Thresholds should be removed in other rooms.
10. A safety gate should be in place at the top of the stairs.
11. A railing should be placed on the right side of the stairs going down.
12. You should not use the back hall, back stairs or back entry to the bathroom.
13. The telephone should be reconnected for emergency use.

We hope you will not mind if we look in on you again in about four to six weeks to see how you are getting along.

SINCERELY

Following discharge, the team makes a follow-up visit after four to six weeks. This is done in an attempt to see how many of the suggestions have actually been followed and to find out whether the patient has maintained his degree of independence, has improved, or has regressed. Even the fact that the family and patient know the team will be in to see him later on is an incentive to keep up the activity which the patient has learned through his rehabilitation training (see Chart 10).

CHART 9

FORM USED AT TIME OF HOME EVALUATION

Name	Sex Age
Address	Adm. Date
Diagnosis	Dis. Date
Attitude of Patient (or Relative)	Hm. Visit Date

Accepted
 Gladly ....
 Reluctantly ....
Refused

  Functional Status at Time of Home Visit
   Explanation

  Deficiency
 (Check if present)
Vision ....
Communication
 Speech ....
 Writing ....
 Hearing ....
Self-Care
 Feeding ....
 Bathing ....
 Dressing ....
 Grooming ....
Locomotion
 Transferring ....
 Wheelchair
  management ....
 Ambulation ....
 Stair climbing ....
Household
 Activities ....
Additional Remarks:

Goals to be achieved before discharge:

In our experience, we have found most families to be very cooperative in following most recommendations. Obviously those suggestions which are most necessary and which involve the patient's comfort are usually taken care of first. These would include such things as proper safety measures, installation of toilet seats, arrangement of furniture in bedrooms, and removal of scatter rugs. Other items which require more major alteration or cash outlay, such as building ramps, putting railings on staircases, etc., are less often accomplished. This is sometimes due to the fact that the family is renting and landlords will not allow major alterations to be done. In some instances, actual change of living quarters has been recommended, and this is also sometimes difficult for a family to accept.

CHART 9 (CONTINUED)

Evaluation of Home or Nursing Home Environment

1. Areas requiring adaptation:
   a. Bedroom

   b. Bathroom

   c. Kitchen

   d. Other living quarters

   e. Floors (thresholds, rugs)

   f. Stairs or elevator (Inside and outside railings)

   g. Other

2. Transportation inadequacies:

3. Clothing and equipment requiring adaptation:

4. Nursing inadequacies and hygiene:

5. Speech therapy, communication needs:

6. Other problems affecting maintenance of rehabilitation goals:

List home visiting team, including students:

Date

CHART 10

<small>FORM USED AT TIME OF FOLLOW-UP VISIT</small>

Name   Sex   Age

Address   Follow-up Visit No.

Diagnosis   Date

Length of Time Since Discharge

    I.   Functional status change at time of discharge.

    II. Summary of post-discharge visit and/or performance.

(Summary should include deficiencies in communication, self-care locomotion and household activities which resulted from failure to follow recommendations.)

Did family physician participate in any way in patient's program?

List home visiting team, including students:

The home evaluation is also very helpful to the staff by filling in a gap in their total knowledge of the patient. They finally get to see the patient as he is going to be functioning within his own family unit. It often reveals that one has pursued unrealistic rehabilitation goals. For instance, much time is spent in training the patient to get in and out of a bathtub independently. When the visit is made, one may find that there is no bathtub, but the patient has not admitted this because he is ashamed to let anyone know that he lived all these years without taking a tub bath.

Upon comparing the abilities of stroke patients who were discharged before the home evaluation program was put into effect with those of patients who have been discharged since, it is obvious that this program made a significant contribution to the overall rehabilitation of the patient. These patients are now able to function more effectively and more safely. They have more confidence and usually maintain or improve their abilities rather than regress.

Chapter XV

THE TEAM AT WORK

A 64-YEAR-OLD MARRIED female, A. B., had prepared for months to visit in another state with her daughter over the Christmas-New Year holidays. She had been relatively well, although she was under the care of her private physician for rheumatic heart disease with mitral and aortic valvular lesions and auricular fibrillation. She had worked very hard in preparation for the trip and finally flew with her husband in late December to make the visit. The day after New Years she was suddenly stricken with paralysis of the right arm and leg and loss of speech. She was seen immediately by her daughter's physician who hospitalized her and administered the immediate treatment for her stroke. Primary attention was paid to the prevention of further embolic phenomenon by giving an anticoagulant.

Contact was made with the chronic disease division of the Department of Health, Education, and Welfare to seek rehabilitation services near her home. It was recommended that the patient be transferred to the Cardinal Cushing Rehabilitation Center. As soon as the acuteness of the illness had passed, the patient was flown from the out-of-state hospital to the Cardinal Cushing Rehabilitation Center accompanied by her husband.

Upon admission to the ward of the rehabilitation center, the patient and her husband were first greeted by the rehabilitation nurse. The nurse made a detailed assessment of the patient's disabilities in order to decide where the patient would be most functional on the ward. It was particularly important to rule out the presence of homonymous hemianopsia because this would involve special placement of the patient in her unit so that her good visual side would be towards the center of activity. It was also important to note the degree of partial aphasia which was

251

present because it was important that an aphasic patient not be placed in a room with other aphasics and thus lack the stimulation of talking to other individuals.

At this time the nurse pointed out to the husband that in this rehabilitation program, the patient would be dressed in her own clothes and usually slacks were to be preferred for women patients because of various physical exercises which they would soon be doing. The husband would also be allowed to bring in a radio or a television set for evening hours if desired. The patient and her husband were then introduced to other patients on the ward and various members of the nursing staff so that she could begin to feel that she was part of the big family with whom she would live for a period of time. The husband was acquainted with the special visiting hours which apply to the rehabilitation center specifically. He was then referred to the social service department for an initial interview and for his first briefing.

The patient's husband was found to be quite anxious about his wife's disability and he had many questions about her needs and various aspects of her treatment. The social worker indicated to him that it was certainly expected that following a comprehensive program the patient would return home and that it was hoped that he would work along as a member of the team in his wife's rehabilitation. The patient was found to be a very gracious, sociable person, but during the first few weeks of the program seemed to reject some of the activities.

The nurses soon after her admission and medical work-up by the house physician, made an assessment of her activity of daily living abilities. They checked her ability to come to a sitting position or get out of bed by herself by transferring on her good leg, and they assessed her abilities in bathing, feeding, dressing, grooming, and tub bathing. She was placed in a standard wheelchair and taught how to manipulate this with her unaffected upper and lower extremities so that she could become mobile on the ward.

She was then presented at the next general evaluation conference and seen by the director of the department who assessed her disability in order to set goals and write the orders for her program. The patient was found to have no voluntary motion in the right upper and lower extremities and a partial expressive aphasia. The goals initially set were to maintain the range of motion of the right upper and lower extremities, to increase the strength of the left upper and lower extremities, to accustom the patient to the upright position and to establish wheelchair independence. To achieve these goals the following orders were written: passive range of motion right upper and lower extremities; progressive resistive exercises left upper and lower extremities; tilt table; wheelchair transfer and mobility. It was noted that should the patient demonstrate a high degree of agility or if return of motion began to occur in the right lower extremity, goals would be upgraded and ambulation possibilities would be considered.

In occupational therapy, treatment was to be directed toward passive range of motion of the right upper extremity and strength and dexterity of the left upper extremity. An activity of daily living check-out was to be done to determine whether any adaptive equipment might be necessary. The patient was to be placed in a group where some speech stimulation would be received.

The patient was also referred to the speech therapist for evaluation and treatment. She was then taken to the various departments for her initial appointments by the nurse whom she had now begun to know and in whom she could feel some security.

Each department made its initial evaluation and recorded measurements which could be used periodically to evaluate actual specific progress. At her first four-week reevaluation, these comparative measurements revealed that the patient was making satisfactory progress. Although she had been disturbed and rejecting during the first few weeks, she had become most cooperative by the last two weeks of the report period except when something new was introduced. She had complained of pain in the left shoulder to extremes of motion, so hot packs were added to her program to help eliminate the discomfort. During the early part of this month the right lower extremity developed voluntary motion in the hip and knee flexors with gravity eliminated as well as hip and knee extension and hip abduction. Dorsiflexion of the ankle was only present in a mass flexion pattern. Because of this active motion it was now possible to begin manual resistive exercises to the right lower extremity. This meant that the patient's prognosis for ambulation now became very good. The upright position in the tilt table was tolerated very rapidly for twenty to thirty minutes and the patient was able to progress to standing in the parallel bars with a posterior splint to stabilize the knee and a temporary assist to stabilize the ankle. She had also very rapidly become wheelchair independent and was able to go to the various departments under her own power.

By the end of this month she was able to walk with the temporary assist outside of the parallel bars using a quad cane, with a fairly acceptable gait, under the close supervision of the therapist. The nurses reported that she was highly motivated towards self-care and had been working specifically on dressing techniques using certain adaptive equipment. She was encouraged to talk as much as possible and words were coming more easily during the last week of the month. Gross motion had returned to the right upper extremity and this was being assisted in occupational therapy by the utilization of a skateboard. Fortunately the patient was ambidextrous and tests revealed that she was quite competent in the use of the left upper extremity. She tested 34 on the gross test for coordination and 6 on the test for fine dexterity. At the end of this month she was independent in all ADL activities except for bathing and putting on her bra.

The speech therapist found that she had limited auditory verbal comprehension for sentences and silent reading comprehension was limited by a tendency to make paraphasic errors. She was unable to perform pretended action but had no difficulty with automatic speech. Written words contained many paraphasic errors and she had difficulty naming parts of the body.

During this period the social service department had worked with the patient's husband, and as the patient improved his anxiety began to lessen. The patient was invited to join a group of female stroke patients being seen in group therapy by the social service worker, and she not only contributed to this program, but received help through this medium of expression and could now agree that her husband had the right idea in arranging for her admission to the rehabilitation center. She was fitted with new glasses which helped her vision, and by the end of six weeks she was ready to leave the hospital and take a look at a new ranchstyle home which was being built for her and her husband.

The patient now made frequent use of the beauty parlor and kept herself in impeccable condition. At the end of eight weeks there was additional significant progress. Pain in the extremes of motion in the right shoulder had diminished; she began to show finger activity and elbow flexion; muscle power in the right lower extremity was improving, and she now had a double upright short-leg brace with Klenzak ankle. She walked to and from the department with supervision and no longer required her wheelchair. Her speech was improving, but she needed constant repetition of some situations from day to day in order to remember.

At the end of ten weeks the patient had reached what appeared to be her maximum level of independence. She now walked independently with a quad cane and managed stairs. There had been continued improvement in her work tolerance and in occupational therapy she was tested out in the kitchen and found able to cook simple foods and wash dishes. She was completely independent in all activities of daily living. The patient lived in an area beyond the limits of the usual evaluation program, but the therapists sat down with the husband and discussed the layout of the new home and it was found that little adapting was required for the patient's limitations. She was discharged at this time to the care of her husband and was expected to make an excellent adjustment in view of her warm, healthy marital relationship.

The patient had made such a close and warm relationship with the hairdresser that follow-up assessments were simplified because the patient returned to the hospital hairdresser to have her hair styled. The patient has continued to live an independent happy life at home and has been most appreciative of the efforts of each member of the team.

Chapter XVI

CONCLUSION

IN THE PREVIOUS chapters an attempt has been made to describe how the rehabilitation team works together to restore the cerebrovascular accident patient to maximum independence. Our concept of the philosophy necessary in the care of this type of patient has been expressed. The special contributions which each member of the team provides have been described and a case presentation has been given to demonstrate how each of these separate services work together to create the final result. It remains then to provide some concrete statistics which substantiate our premise that the basic concept of this book is justifiable and that if this approach is used, the stroke patient has a significant chance to return to the community as a fairly independent individual.

Mahoney *et al.*, in 1955, reported results of two surveys made in a large veteran's administration hospital. In the first study of 122 inpatients, 81.8 per cent reached independence at the time of discharge. In the second study of 70 patients, 71.9 per cent reached independence in ambulation before discharge, while an additional 17.1 per cent attained safe and independent self-care while remaining confined to wheelchairs. In 1962, Barrow summarized the literature showing that early ambulation, encouragement of independent activity, and regular persistent physical therapy shortened hospitalization and improved return of functional activity. Most patients became independent and 10 to 15 per cent returned to some form of gainful employment. We recently compiled statistics concerning 380 unselected stroke patients treated in the rehabilitation program at the Cardinal Cushing Rehabilitation Center, Holy Ghost Hospital, Cambridge, Massachusetts. The severity of their disability ranged from the total hemiplegic with complete motor aphasia, to the hemiparetic with little residual difficulty. The main criterion for admission to the program was the ability of the patient to follow simple commands and to cooperate in an active program. Mild to moderate mental confusion or memory defect did not disqualify the patient from participation. The specific rehabilitation program was adapted to each patient's needs and consisted of the conventional method of the team approach which has been presented in the foregoing chapters. Inpatients were considered successful attaining either complete independence or independence with supervision and/or mild assistance of a degree permitting discharge from the hospital and return into the community. This independence could be either in ambulation or in wheelchair mobility, plus competence in the activities of daily living (ADL). The discharges were to patients' own homes, relatives' homes, or to boarding or nursing homes if the former were not available.

Outpatients (already ambulatory and usually independent in ADL) were considered successful if they reached the specific goals set for them at evaluation. These goals varied depending upon initial residual disability. Of the 380 unselected cases, 293, or 77.1 per cent were classified as successful; 246 of these were inpatients and 47 were outpatients. The remainder of this chapter will describe the ADL results obtained in the 246 successful inpatients.

Certain quantitative criteria were established in order to express comparatively the initial status, the discharge status, and the status at follow-up whenever possible. These criteria were kept simple, yet specific enough for measurement of progress. The degrees of independence in the various areas studied were graded from one to three. Stage one indicated complete independence; stage two, partial dependence at three different levels; and stage three, heavy dependence upon the assistance of others (see Chap. VII, Charts 4-8).

As most patients referred for physical therapy had unfortunately been bedridden for significant periods of time, manipulating a wheelchair was the initial step towards mobilization. This did allow freedom of movement around the ward. The technique of managing a wheelchair with one arm or leg was not always simple. However 91 per cent of the patients were dependent upon admission in this category, and 95 per cent of these patients achieved either complete independence or were included in the two top levels of partial dependence. Most patients wished to be mobile and the motivation to master this technique was high.

Dressing and grooming, bathing, tub bathing, toileting, and feeding were included on one assessment sheet. In order to confine as much information as possible to one sheet, the specific level of ability was encircled in red upon admission, in black upon discharge, and in green at the time of follow-up.

Sixty-three per cent of the patients were completely dependent in dressing upon admission; 88 per cent achieved either complete independence or were included in the two top levels of partial dependence. The greatest problems were seen with patients left with a functionless upper and lower extremity in an activity such as putting the brace, the shoe, and the stocking on the affected lower extremity. Most patients enjoyed being able to dress in their own clothing and related well in most instances to the tedious teaching process and to the use of adaptive equipment.

Sixty-three per cent of the patients were completely dependent in simple bathing, and 89 per cent achieved complete independence or were included in the two top levels of partial dependence. Again, most patients enjoyed being able to accomplish this activity with some privacy. The patient with one functionless upper extremity had difficulty in bathing the non-affected upper extremity and distal portions of the body.

Ninety-two per cent of the patients were unable to use the tub, and only 71 per cent achieved success. However, it was found many patients regressed in this activity upon going home. Many of these older patients had not been regular users of the tub even before their disability. This appeared to be an activity inspiring a much lower motivation.

Eighty-four per cent of patients were completely dependent in toilet activity. This also appeared to inspire high motivation as 89 per cent of the patients achieved independence with or without toilet aids.

Only 13 per cent of these patients were completely dependent in feeding, and 99 per cent achieved complete independence or were included in the two top levels of partial dependence. This was a high motivation, simpler activity, and in fact, many of the dependent 13 per cent were only in this category because they had not been allowed to feed themselves while in general hospitals. This accentuated the role many general hospital personnel play in fostering dependency in disabled patients.

Eighty-three per cent of patients were completely dependent in ambulation upon admission, and 86 per cent achieved independence or were included in the two top levels of partial dependence. This included some patients with plegic lower extremities who required long-leg braces.

It is therefore our feeling that all stroke patients who are mentally alert and can follow simple commands deserve a trial at rehabilitation therapy. The majority will have a successful experience and if physical restoration is not total, the general condition and health of these patients will at least be improved. It is the sincere hope of the authors that the material presented in this book will be helpful to the practicing physician in the everyday care of his patient. General hospitals must become much more invested in the care of the stroke patient and set up special stroke programs so that early mobilization, preservation of function, and prevention of complications is accomplished. The patient who then needs further rehabilitation should be rapidly referred to the team of specialists who can best perform the physical restoration procedures. In this way the best possible comprehensive medicine will finally reach down to the stroke patient—currently a most neglected member of our society.

REFERENCES

BARROW, J. G.; CARY, F. H., AND GAHIMER, J. E.: Development of a stroke program in Georgia. *Amer J Public Health*, 52:627, 1962.

BONNER, C. D., AND NELSON, A. H.: Results of physical rehabilitation in 380 patients with cerebral vascular accidents. *Proc. First Caribbean Congr in Phys Med Rehab*, 1:131, 1966.

MAHONEY, F. L.; BARTHEL, D. W., AND CALLAHAN, J. P.: Rehabilitation of the hemiplegic patient: A clinical evaluation. *Southern Med J*, 48:472, 1955.

INDEX